M000251754

Upper Cervical Practice Mastery

Learn Success Secrets of the World's Top Upper Cervical Doctors

Dr. Bill Davis

Copyright © 2018 Dr. Bill Davis

All rights reserved.

ISBN-10: 0692154558
ISBN-13: 978-0692154557

DEDICATION

This book is dedicated to God, my wife Julie, my kids Ethan, Isaac, and Grace, our team at Upper Cervical Marketing, sick and suffering people looking for hope and healing, and all of the excellent Upper Cervical Doctors and future Doctors around the world.

CONTENTS

ACKNOWLEDGMENTS

I want to thank my wife Julie Davis for her great contribution to this book. I want to thank our team at Upper Cervical Marketing including Heather Compton, Tony Hook, Summer Grohman, Jhon Arellano, Joemar Garraton, Jiesie Lota, Chris Dayagdag, Dr. Jane Brewer, Adam Kantrowitz, Jessica Zamora, Patti Lougee, Stephanie Radan, Kelly Allen, Clare O'Brien, and Erbe Garchitorena for their contributions. I also want to thank all of the top Upper Cervical Doctors, Coaches, and Advocates that I have interviewed or I have featured in this book including Dr. Jeff Scholten, Dr. Terry McCoskey, Dr. Larry Arbeitman, Dr. Jamie Cramer, Dr. Todd Osborne, Dr. Dennis Young, Dr. Andy Gibson, Dr. Ian Davis-Tremayne, Dr. Kerry Johnson, Dr. Noel Lloyd, Dr. Robert Brooks, Dr. Corinne Weaver, Keith Wassung, Dr. Michael Lenarz, Dr. Christine Zapata, Dr. Steve Judson, Dr. Julie Mayer-Hunt, Dr. Ed Gigliotti, Dr. Justin Brown, Dr. Kurt Sherwood, Dr. Christina Meakim, Dr. Drew Hall, Dr. Jon Baker, James Tomasi, Dr. Giancarlo Licata, Dr. Shawn Dill, Dr. Ian Bulow, Dr. Christopher Perkins, Dr. Joe Breuwet, Dr. Brett Gottlieb, Dr. Casey Weerheim, Dr. Kristen McClure, Dr. Geoff Besso, Dr. Benjamin Kuhn, Dr. Kyrie Kleinfelter, and Dr. Miguel Flores. Your commitment to excellence in bringing hope and healing to sick and suffering people is an inspiration to me every day.

INTRODUCTION

I decided to write this book because I love Upper Cervical Chiropractic and I want people all over the world to have access to this incredible type of care.

But unfortunately, without thriving Upper Cervical Practices all over the world, this dream is impossible.

Up to this point, there has not been a book that specifically focuses on Upper Cervical Practices and the unique challenges and opportunities that Upper Cervical Doctors have.

In 2008 after an associate position I went on my own starting an Upper Cervical Practice in Southern California and I wish I had a resource like this in my hands to guide me before and during the launch of my first Upper Cervical Practice.

It is only by the grace of God that I was able to build an all-cash $30,000 per month Upper Cervical Practice from scratch in only three years.

In November of 2011 while mountain biking with some friends I suffered a spinal cord injury and was paralyzed. Unfortunately, I have been unable to practice since then.

But in 2013 God revealed to me a new plan and purpose he had for my life and that was to start Upper Cervical Marketing to help Upper Cervical Doctors and students thrive in practice. This book is a logical next step in accomplishing this purpose.

Over the past five years, I have personally worked with over 200 Upper Cervical Practices and have interviewed nearly 100 more of the top Upper Cervical Doctors in our profession on The Upper Cervical Marketing Podcast. It is with this experience that I wrote this book to help you master Upper Cervical Practice and grow Upper Cervical in your community and around the world.

Survey Says!

Since 2015 our Upper Cervical Marketing Team has been doing an annual Upper Cervical Practice Survey and have discovered some startling statistics from the 659 Upper Cervical Practices we have surveyed:

- **19% of doctors are collecting less than $10,000 per month**
- **45% of doctors are collecting less than $20,000 per month**
- **13% of doctors see less than 50 patient visits per week**
- **74% of doctors are in solo practice**
- **36% of doctors number one problem is generating enough new patients**
- **10% of doctors see 5 new patients or less per month**

Once I was aware of how many Doctors are struggling and realized that many of them just don't know what they don't know, I knew I had to do something. I wanted to share all the wisdom I have learned from the top Upper Cervical Doctors in our profession as well as my own experience in building a $30,000 per month Upper Cervical Practice in three years and now a $1 million online marketing agency in five years.

First, let's answer some questions that might be on your mind.

Who is this book for?

This book is written with several different groups in mind including:

- Chiropractic students who want to thrive in their first year of practice
- New practice owners who want to learn from the best
- Established but struggling doctors who finally want to get their head above water
- Thriving doctors who want to continue to grow and take their practice to the next level

Will the principles in this book work for cash practices only?

While I personally believe that Upper Cervical Practices should be all cash in almost every circumstance, the principles in this book will work for insurance practices as well.

Will the principles in this book work for all Upper Cervical Techniques?

Yes if you are an Upper Cervical Practitioner you can be extremely successful in practice regardless of your technique if you apply the principles in this book.

How is Upper Cervical Practice Mastery structured?

The book is set up sequentially, meaning that the chapters at the beginning are vital to master before focusing on the middle chapters and the later chapters.

How do you use it?

How you use this book will depend on your current situation.

- If you are a chiropractic student or new practice owner start from chapter 1 and go chapter by chapter applying the principles and habits along the way to set yourself up for success.

- If you are an established but struggling Doc, start from the beginning and work your way through, making sure to really focus on the first section. In my experience, this is the section that most Doctors who are failing are struggling with the most. You may even want to read the first section several times before moving on to the other sections.

- If you are a thriving Doc who wants to continue to grow, you could read specific chapters that are the most interesting to you or that focus on areas that you know you need to work on. However, reading it through from the beginning may be a great encouragement to you as you recognize all the things you have done correctly to get you where you are today and hopefully inspire you to keep growing.

I hope as you read this book it will make a dramatic impact on your life and you too can become an Upper Cervical Practice Master with an extraordinary practice.

SECTION 1: PERSONAL MASTERY

"You are what you are and where you are because of what has gone into your mind. You can change what you are and where you are by changing what goes into your mind."

– Zig Ziglar

CHAPTER ONE

EVALUATE YOUR LIFE

The 10 Life Domains

"The unexamined life is not worth living"

— Socrates

How you do anything is how you do everything.

This is a phrase that is very true in many ways.

Your practice is a direct reflection of your life.

- If you're building a house…your practice will be affected.

- If you have a child that is struggling with drugs…your practice will be affected.

- If you are going through a divorce…your practice will be affected.

- If you have a health crisis…your practice will be affected.

If your life is in chaos your practice will be in chaos.

This is why it's so important that we discuss personal mastery before we can discuss practice mastery or growth mastery.

Without a commitment to taking ownership and growing in all areas of your life, your practice will never be as great as it can be.

If you don't have integrity in your personal life you likely won't have integrity in your practice.

Integrity by definition is a wholeness.

This is where we get the word integer, and integers are whole numbers.

When you have integrity or wholeness in all areas of your life your practice will be more likely to grow.

The top Upper Cervical Doctors have a strong self-awareness and are able to evaluate themselves and consistently improve.

10 LIFE DOMAINS

A tremendous tool for developing self-awareness is to look at your 10 life domains.

Your life consists of Ten Life Domains

1. **Spiritual**
2. **Intellectual**
3. **Emotional**
4. **Physical**
5. **Marital**
6. **Parental**
7. **Social**
8. **Vocational**
9. **Avocational**
10. **Financial**

Michael Hyatt has a great tool called the Life Score Assessment that I use on a weekly basis to determine where I am in these 10 life domains. The life score assessment allows you to rate yourself on a score of 1 to 12 in each of the 10 life domains.

You can get Michael Hyatt's life score assessment at https://assessments.michaelhyatt.com/lifescore/.

I'm going to discuss each of the domains and what the highest and lowest score is in each dimension. **<u>As I go through these think about how you would rate yourself at this time in your life.</u>**

Determine for yourself if there is a particular domain in which you are struggling.

SPIRITUAL

The spiritual domain of your life has the greatest impact on all the other domains.

1 = I feel disconnected from God. I am not taking any initiative to pursue spiritual development. I feel rudderless and wonder if my life even matters. I am not part of any faith community.

12 = I am constantly aware of God's presence in my life. I am consistent in my spiritual disciplines. I am clear about my purpose and how it relates to God's larger story. I'm a contributing leader in my faith community.

INTELLECTUAL

Your intellectual domain comes down to how well you nurture and cultivate your mind.

1 = I am content with what I know and am not interested in growing further. I don't regularly consume new content. I don't attend conferences or workshops. I don't allocate any money for ongoing education or training.

12 = I am a voracious learner. I can't seem to get enough new content. I am a conference and workshop junkie. I highly value ongoing education and consider each expense an investment.

EMOTIONAL

Your emotional domain is focused on how much you allow your life circumstances to impact your moods.

1 = I am often sad and don't have much energy. I struggle with low self-esteem and worry. I am often stressed and use alcohol, drugs, or other addictive behaviors to deal with it. I often find myself angry and resentful of others.

12 = I am almost always happy. I am confident and optimistic about the future. I don't experience any significant stress. I empathize with other's struggles and shortcomings.

PHYSICAL

Your physical state is how your body functions and feels.

1 = I am usually tired and feel lethargic. I eat too much sugar and processed food. I don't take any supplements. I do not exercise regularly.

12 = I see my body as a gift and consistently make healthy choices to take care of it. I wake up well rested. I eat a balanced diet of unprocessed, organic food. I have a dialed-in, consistent fitness routine that gives me energy and strength. Unhealthy behaviors are rarely if ever, a temptation.

MARITAL

Your spouse can be your greatest strength or your greatest weakness. If you are not currently married then you would skip this section.

1 = I am no longer in love with my spouse and am considering divorce. I can hardly stand to be in the same room with my spouse. I am frustrated with my spouse and don't understand why he/she can't change. We experience a lot of conflict and continue to drift further and further apart.

12 = I love my spouse more with each passing day. My spouse and I tell each other everything and actively seek one another's counsel. My spouse and I want our marriage to be the best it can possibly be and invest in making it better. We experience little conflict because we seek first to understand rather than to be understood.

PARENTAL

Your parental domain is focused on your relationship with your kids. If you do not currently have children then you would again skip this section.

1 = I don't really enjoy being a parent. If I am honest, wish I had never had children. I don't feel prepared to be a parent. My children are a major source of conflict and stress.

12 = I love being a parent and know it's my most important work. I love my children and enjoy spending time with them. My children feel comfortable sharing their deepest desires and greatest fears. When we experience conflict, we resolve it in a way that leads to greater intimacy.

SOCIAL

Your social domain is the state of the friendships in your life.

1 = I don't have a best friend. I don't have any friends outside of work. I often feel lonely and spend my time online, watching TV, or indulging in unhealthy behavior. Many of my past friendships have ended over unresolved conflict.

12 = I have a best friend with whom I can share my biggest dreams and my greatest fears. I have a close circle of friends with whom I "do life." I can't wait to spend time with my friends. My relationships are one of my greatest sources of joy. When we experience conflict, we resolve it in a way that leads to greater intimacy.

VOCATIONAL

Your vocational domain is how you see your work.

1 = I hate my job and wish I could find something else to do. I dread going to work and live for the weekends. I feel like I am going backward in my vocation. I am not happy with my level of income.

12 = I love my work and am confident I am making a big impact in the world. I am at the top of my game and am the recognized leader in my industry. I am growing faster than I ever thought possible and find the pace exhilarating. I am making more money than I need and love having the margin to invest in the future and in worthy causes.

AVOCATIONAL

This is your hobbies and other pursuits that you enjoy.

1 = I don't have time to pursue interests outside of work and family. I don't have any hobbies nor do I have the time if I did. I am not involved in any significant way in civic or church activities. My life consists of work and family—that's pretty much it.

12 = I have all the time I need to pursue interests outside of work. I have a hobby that I could probably turn into a vocation if I wanted. I have a group of fellow-enthusiasts that I enjoy spending time within the pursuit of our hobby. I am involved in a leadership role in a non-profit charity, school, or ministry that is changing the world.

FINANCIAL

This is your ability to make money, spend money, save money and give money. Are you wise or are you foolish?

1 = I worry constantly about my finances and am fearful about the future. I do not make enough money to cover my family's basic needs. I am not really saving anything for retirement—or anything else. I am deeply in debt and don't currently see a way out.

12 = I rarely think about my finances because I have all the bases covered. I make more than enough money for my needs and am able to give generously to causes that matter. I don't have any debt, not even a mortgage. My net worth is more than I could have imagined a few years ago and feel it will continue to grow.

Assessing yourself in these 10 life domains will give you the ability to see the areas of your life that are holding you back from having an extraordinary and abundant life.

Once you identify the areas that you would score low, you can then put a plan in place to improve these areas. Many of these areas will not change quickly but will take commitment and consistency in your habits. We will talk more about that in the next two chapters.

If you have rated yourself in the "Danger Zone" (scores of 1 to 3) in any of these domains it is crucial that you begin making changes immediately.

You should focus on the domain(s) in danger by making intentional deposits. Chances are these low scoring domains are already affecting other higher scoring domains so you will need to be swift in your approach to bring your score(s) up out of the danger zone.

THE MYTH OF WORK-LIFE BALANCE

Myth: Every week of your work and personal life should be perfectly balanced.

It is important to understand that your life may not be in perfect balance during every season you are in practice. There will be weeks, sometimes months that you will need to work long hours. However, there will also be some weeks where you will find yourself working much less.

In episode 48 of the Upper Cervical Marketing podcast, Dr. Christine Zapata and I discuss how she invested long hours and sweat equity when her practice was first beginning. It was only after many years of focused intensity that she was able to achieve the life balance that she has now.

Having realistic expectations for achieving your own life balance will help you keep the process in perspective.

If you just started your practice then it's completely reasonable for you to be working more now than you ever have.

If you have a family, they can deal with an intense work schedule for a season. If there is a goal in sight of greater family time and financial rewards, even small children can endure stretches of time when one parent is not as present.

Just be sure that the time you do spend with your family in this busy work season is quality time. However, if you continue to ask your family to wait while you pursue all of your practice dreams, don't be surprised if they seem more distant and your relationship with each member suffers. If you focus so much on your practice dreams and don't keep it balanced with your family and their dreams, you may lose them altogether.

A lack of balance for years or decades is not a good approach to building a successful practice. Your goal should be to build a successful practice while also building a successful family life.

If you don't have a family yet, this is a great time to really focus on building your dream practice before you settle down, however, balance is still important. Make time for yourself, be intentional about having a social life and stay active in your faith. Then, if and when a family does come into the picture, you will have a good routine of balance already established.

Likewise, if you put your health on hold for too long eventually you will get sick. Don't neglect your personal health and well-being while you pursue your practice goals. Rather, incorporate your health goals into your practice goals. You will be of no use to your patients or staff if you are sick and unable to give them your best.

In the next chapter, we will discuss the mindset that is necessary to have the personal mastery that will lead to abundance in your life and practice.

CHAPTER TWO

BUILD A MINDSET THAT WINS

The 7 Characteristics of a Winning Mindset

"All of life is peaks and valleys.
Don't let the peaks get too high or the
valleys too low."

– John Wooden

On November 25, 2011, I had a thriving all-cash Upper Cervical Practice collecting $30,000 per month and I had a mindset that was winning.

The next morning, I went mountain biking with some friends and everything changed.

I flipped over on my mountain bike while traveling at high-speed downhill and suffered a C7 burst fracture and spinal cord injury.

The paralysis that came with the spinal cord injury made it impossible for me to stand, walk or use my left hand and my right hand has limited function.

I also have many other issues with organ function that limit my daily activities. I spent the next three months in the hospital recovering from my injuries and when I left in a wheelchair and made my way back to my practice over 80% of my practice was gone.

It took me time to realize that my mindset was dramatically impacted by my injuries and it took me years to get back that winning mindset.

Using my own experience and knowledge gathered from interviews with some of the top Upper Cervical Chiropractors in our profession (featured on the UCM Podcast), I have been able to identify 7 characteristics of a winning mindset.

These characteristics help to cultivate and focus your mind on the things that matter the most which free you from anything that is not essential to a winning mindset.

PURPOSE

Ralph Waldo Emerson said:

> *"The purpose of life is not to be happy. It is to be useful, to be honorable, to be compassionate, to have it make some difference that you have lived and lived well."*

One of the most important aspects of recovery from a major life event like paralysis is finding a renewed purpose, a new why.

If you have suffered a major life event such as:
- injury or illness
- divorce
- death of a loved one
- failure of a business

It is important that you also find a renewed purpose.

Regardless of whether or not you have suffered a major life event, the fact remains that PURPOSE is the driving force behind all of the top Upper Cervical Doctors that I know.

In episode 47 Dr. Steve Judson and I discussed the importance of purpose as a driving force in developing his Upper Cervical Practice to over 1000 visits per week. His purpose is focused on helping those with mental illness find recovery and health through upper cervical chiropractic.

In episode 10 I also discussed the importance of purpose with Dr. Julie Mayer-Hunt whose powerful purpose began with her father and is now being carried on by herself and her son as well. This generational purpose has allowed her to help develop the Upper Cervical Diplomate and she is now leaving a legacy for Upper Cervical Chiropractors throughout the world.

I found my purpose again when I began writing blog posts for a friend in March of 2013.

After having to close my practice I was able to see a renewed purpose and focus in helping other Upper Cervical Doctors throughout the world reach sick and suffering people in their community through the power of the Internet.

Over the past five years, we have helped hundreds of doctors reach over 20,000 new patients with the upper cervical message through our Upper Cervical Marketing System.

What about you?

To determine your own purpose think through these questions:
- Why are you here?
- Why did God put you on this earth?
- How can you make a powerful impact in your community?
- How can you leave a legacy?
- How can you change the way people think about health?

Starting to determine your own personal purpose and philosophy will allow you to keep your mind focused on your purpose even when your journey to practice mastery has challenges…which it most definitely will.

INTENTIONALITY

Once your mind is focused on your purpose the next characteristic to focus on is having intentionality.

Intentionality is defined as "being **deliberate or purposive**."

Intentionality is taking your purpose and applying your daily thought patterns and activities deliberately to living out your purpose.

I discussed this with Dr. Ed Gigliotti in episode 44 when he talked about how his practice was struggling until he was able to define his purpose and become extremely intentional in his day-to-day thought patterns and communication. Jesus said in Luke 6:45:

"out of the abundance of the heart the mouth speaks"

When your purpose is driving you and you are deliberate in your thought patterns than your mouth will speak that which is in your heart.

CONFIDENCE

When your purpose is crystal clear and your thought patterns are deliberate and intentional then your communication to patients and your team will be with confidence and certainty.

I spoke about this several times with Dr. Justin Brown on episode 15. Dr. Brown has one of the largest Upper Cervical Practices in the world and has built his spectacular practice in an incredibly short period of time.

Dr. Brown has a powerful purpose and is extremely intentional in how he lives his life and as a result of that when you speak with him he speaks with confidence, certainty, and authority. This is a powerful combination.

If your confidence is shot and you are struggling to communicate with certainty and authority to your patients then go back and re-examine your purpose. Define your purpose very clearly to yourself and then become intentional and deliberate day-by-day, hour-by-hour and moment-by-moment to reinforce your purpose to yourself.

Read your success stories, remind yourself of the ways you have helped patients' lives change. It is easy to get discouraged in chiropractic practice and this can lead to ineffective doctors who lack confidence. Go back to your purpose, focus on developing those intentional thought patterns and your confidence will begin to grow.

PATIENCE

Patience is possibly the most difficult of all 7 of the characteristics of a mindset that wins.

In our instant digital world, we get frustrated if a website doesn't load in three seconds. This can make it difficult to be patient with ourselves and our practice.

Success in practice and in life is a journey, not a destination. There will always be an area of your practice or your personal life that is not where you want them to be. Most likely, you will be unhappy with several areas at the same time so having patience is key.

In Jim Collins' fantastic business book ***Good to Great*** he discusses the Stockdale Paradox. The Stockdale Paradox is named after Admiral Jim Stockdale, who was the highest ranking United States military officer held captive for eight years during the Vietnam War. Stockdale was tortured more than twenty times by his captors, and never had much reason to believe he would survive the POW camp. And yet, as Stockdale told Collins, he never lost faith during his ordeal:

> *"I never doubted not only that I would get out, but also that I would prevail in the end and turn the experience into the defining event of my life, which, in retrospect, I would not trade."*

Then comes the paradox.

While Stockdale had remarkable faith in the unknowable, he noted that it was always the most optimistic of his prison mates who failed to make it out of there alive.

> *"They were the ones who said, 'We're going to be out by Christmas.' And Christmas would come, and Christmas would go. Then they'd say, 'We're going to be out by Easter.' And Easter would come, and Easter would go. And then Thanksgiving, and then it would be Christmas again. And they died of a broken heart."*

What the optimists failed to do was confront the reality of their situation.

They preferred the ostrich approach, sticking their heads in the sand and hoping for the difficulties to go away. That self-delusion might have made it easier on them in the short-term, but when they were eventually forced to face reality, it had become too much and they couldn't handle it.

Stockdale approached adversity with a very different mindset.

He accepted the reality of his situation, but, rather than bury his head in the sand, he stepped up and did everything he could to lift the morale and prolong the lives of his fellow prisoners. He created a tapping code so they could communicate with each other. He developed a milestone system that helped them deal with torture. And he sent intelligence information to his wife, hidden in the seemingly innocent letters he wrote.

For me, the Stockdale Paradox carries an important lesson in personal development, a lesson in patience, faith, and honesty:

Never doubt that you can achieve your goals, no matter how lofty they may be and no matter how many critics and naysayers you may have. But at the same time, always take honest stock of your current situation. Don't lie to yourself for fear of short-term embarrassment or discomfort, because such deception will only come back to defeat you in the end.

You will need to embrace the second half of the Stockdale Paradox to really make strides. You must **combine that optimism with brutal honesty and a willingness to take action**.

Patience is not the same as complacency.

Admit the truth of your current situation and then **get to work** on improving your situation while at the same time believing that you will prevail in the end.

Many times, we struggle to have patience because we are comparing our beginning to a colleague's middle or our middle to someone else's end.

Enjoy where you are.

Do your best to improve yourself and your practice each day and you will be amazed at what you can accomplish.

PERSEVERANCE

When I left my associate position in 2008 I moved my family to the San Diego area, had our third child, and opened a practice all within eight weeks!

It was an absolute whirlwind.

As an associate, you have no idea how difficult practice can be. Instead most the time you think you can do it a whole lot better than your clinic director and can't wait to get out on your own.

That was my situation and exactly what I was thinking. After two years in my associate position, I could not wait to get my own practice going. When I opened in May 2008 in a new city with no patients I was in a desperate situation.

My wife was at home with the three kids ages 3 1/2 and under I had over ¼ million dollars' worth of debt and no idea how I was going to make my practice work.

I don't recommend putting yourself in this situation but for me, it lit a fire under me like nothing else could. I was working with AMC, a chiropractic management company in their Right Start Program and they helped me tremendously with my initial marketing plan and patient communication.

However, even with that baseline of knowledge, I started every day on my knees praying and crying out to God for His help.

By my third month in practice, I collected $16,000 in one month and thought after that it would all just be easy going.

Boy was I wrong.

I continued to struggle and learn the hard way how to succeed in practice.

I worked hard to learn all that I could from AMC and also about my technique NUCCA.

In my first year I went to 10 technique and practice management seminars, 2 NUCCA conferences, 2 Dr. Albert Berti NUCCA Seminars and 6 AMC Boot Camps.

It was during these early years in practice that I had to learn the lessons of perseverance and persistence.

After my injury in 2011, I once again had to apply what I'd learned in the past and learn a whole different level of perseverance and persistence to do the most basic things in life.

My story is consistent with many others including Dr. Kurt Sherwood who discussed with me in episode 37 about his success in practice through consistent and persistent action and perseverance.

When you combine a focused purpose, intentional and deliberate thought patterns, confident communication to yourself and others, and patience with perseverance and persistence you are getting closer and closer to that winning mindset.

HUMILITY

Humility is a difficult characteristic to talk about.

As the Zig Ziglar saying goes...

> **"Have you heard about the man who received a badge for humility and they had to take it away from him because he wore it"**

Or as the song goes...(to the tune of "If you're happy and you know it, clap your hands")

"If you're humble and you know it...no you're not"

Jesus said it best, as usual in Matthew 23:12:

> **"Whoever exalts himself will be humbled and whoever humbles himself will be exalted"**

Humility is a crucial part of a winner's mindset.

When most people think about having a lack of humility they think of arrogance or boastful pride.

Yet there is another type of pride that is often mislabeled, it's called self-pity. Arrogance and self-pity are definitely on opposite ends of the pride spectrum, but they are both all about self.

Humility, however, is about putting your focus on others and taking it off of self or being self-LESS.

CS Lewis said:

> **"Humility is not thinking less of yourself it is thinking of yourself less"**

If you are struggling in practice it's very likely that you are in a place of self-pity. You really have to break out of that.

By focusing on what you can do today to make your situation better you can begin to gain some control over your life.

If you are successful in practice there is another more insidious way that a lack of humility will impact you and your practice and that is called the arrogance of success.

William Pollard once said:

> *"Learning and innovation go hand in hand. The arrogance of success is to think that what you did yesterday will be sufficient for tomorrow."*

When we reach a certain level of success we can become filled up with pride and arrogance.

A humble person knows that they have never arrived.

There is always more to learn.

Someone who is filled with arrogance can become greedy and forget the importance of giving to others, including their team members.

When we don't share our successes with our team as they happen, over time, resentment will begin to take root within your team.

Take care of your team and they will take care of your patients.

ENTHUSIASM

Winston Churchill said...

> *"Success is going from one failure to another without losing enthusiasm."*

Enthusiasm is another crucial component of the top Upper Cervical Doctors' mindset. Many doctors have talked about the importance of their enthusiasm, energy, and passion with me in interviews, including Dr. Terry McCoskey, Dr. Christina Meakim, and Dr. Drew Hall.

If you're not enthusiastic about what you're doing, if you're not having fun in practice and if you're not passionate about your purpose, then you might be in the wrong profession.

Or maybe you just need to be reminded.

You have the opportunity to change someone's life forever.

Upper Cervical Chiropractors make a dramatic impact on individuals, families, and their community.

Don't ever take this for granted.

If you have lost your enthusiasm and you need to restore your passion here are some questions to ask yourself:

- Do you remember why you started in this work?
  - o It always goes back to your purpose
- Are you attracting the right types of patients that ENERGIZE you and your practice?
  - o If not, we will show you how to do this later in this book
- Is your team passionate about your mission?
  - o If they don't "get it" you will feel like you're constantly pushing them uphill. This is usually a leadership issue. It's your responsibility to communicate the mission, vision and core values of the company on an ongoing basis. We will talk more about this later.
- Have you stopped doing the things you did to be successful in the first place?
  - o For instance, you used to do progress exams with your patients on a regular basis but now you don't do them at all.
  - o Or you used to do team meetings on a weekly basis but now you only do them when you have major problems within the office.
  - o Or you had a very effective marketing program that was consistently generating new patients, increasing referrals and improving retention and re-activations and you stopped doing it to save money.

Why does this happen?

Frequently, when we are pushing hard to accomplish a particular goal or a certain level of success in anything, once we reach that predetermined level it's within our nature to want to relax.

I've heard doctors say it before this way...

"Sometimes I wish I could just take my foot off the gas for a while."

The truth is in an Upper Cervical Practice and life there is no status quo.

Your practice is either growing or dying.

Either increasing or decreasing.

In practice and in life we should always seek to be growing.

When you find systems, procedures, marketing etc. that works for your practice **KEEP DOING IT.**

When you stop doing the things that made you successful in the first place, you won't be for successful for long.

RESOURCES AND PLAN OF ACTION TO PROMOTE A WINNERS MINDSET

To review the 7 characteristics of a top doctors winning mindset are:

1. **Purpose**
2. **Intentionality**
3. **Confidence**
4. **Patience**
5. **Perseverance**
6. **Humility**
7. **Enthusiasm**

You cannot put this type of mindset on autopilot.

You have to consistently take captive your thoughts and protect your mind to stay focused.

Some of the best ways you can do this are to consistently put good information into your mind including great books, podcasts, and videos.

The best-selling book of all time is the Bible and for good reason.

The Bible will give you an in-depth understanding of who God is and who you are. Packed full of wisdom, history, and understanding that is impossible to get anywhere else.

If you have never read the Bible I strongly encourage you to do so. I would recommend starting with the Gospel of John.

But there are a ton of books within the Bible that are full of wisdom to help you grow personally and professionally including:

Proverbs	Ecclesiastes
Psalms	James
Luke	Mark
Acts	Matthew
1 Timothy	2 Timothy
Colossians	Ephesians
Galatians	Philippians
Nehemiah	Titus

Learn from the wisdom of the Bible, it can make all the difference in your life.

Other Books that help you cultivate a winning mindset:

- Good to Great by Jim Collins
- E Myth Revisited by Michael Gerber
- Traction by Gino Wickman
- Entreleadership by Dave Ramsey
- David and Goliath: Underdogs, Misfits and the Art of Battling Giants by Malcolm Gladwell
- How to Win Friends and Influence People by Dale Carnegie
- The Tipping Point by Malcolm Gladwell
- Great by Choice by Jim Collins
- Business for the Glory of God by Wayne Grudem
- Tribes by Seth Godin
- Outliers by Malcolm Gladwell
- The Go-Giver by Bob Burg
- Getting Things Done by David Allen
- Humility: True Greatness by CJ Mahaney

Podcasts that will help you cultivate a winning mindset:

- The Upper Cervical Marketing Podcast

- EntreLeadership podcast
- Zig Ziglar Podcast

I recommend getting a subscription to audible and getting these books on audio and make sure whenever you're driving or exercising that you're redeeming the time you have been given. Use the time to continually cultivate that winning mindset through the books and podcasts I mentioned above.

Another way to build a mindset that wins is through accountability. We have a companion course that goes along with this ***Upper Cervical Practice Mastery*** book to help you have accountability to the implementation and application of the principles and practices in this book.

To learn more about the companion course go to
http://uppercervicalpracticemastery.com/academy

CHAPTER THREE

CULTIVATE YOUR HABITS

10 Winning Habits That Require Zero Talent but Most Doctors Won't Do

*"We are what we repeatedly do.
Excellence, then, is not an act, but a habit."*

— Aristotle

As you begin this chapter, you should have already taken some time to evaluate your life and have an understanding of the components of a winning mindset for a top Upper Cervical Doctor.

The next step is to begin to build habits into your daily routine that will serve your family, your team, your patients, your community, and you personally.

Several years ago I read about the 10 habits that require zero talent but most people won't do and I realized that these habits were consistent with what top Upper Cervical Doctors were consistently doing.

So as you read through these habits be honest with yourself and identify the ones that may be holding you back the most and focus on developing those habits first.

BEING ON TIME

When you and your team are on time whether it be for your patients or for each other it can make a tremendous difference in the health of your organization.

When you are on time it says to the person that they matter to you.

That their time matters to you.

When your team is on time it says that their work matters to them.

When do you arrive at your office?

Are you the first one there?

Or are you getting there five minutes before your first patient or even later?

Your morning routine can have a dramatic impact on the efficiency and effectiveness of your day. I recommend arriving at your practice at least 15 to 30 minutes before any of your team members and at least 45 minutes to an hour before your first patient.

Try to be mindful of what a patient sees when they come to your office. I always parked away from my building leaving as many parking spaces close to my office available for my patients as possible. As I walked from my parking spot toward my office building I would look at the parking lot and make sure there was nothing that may cause a negative impression in the mind of a new or existing patient. If there was trash I would pick it up. If I noticed anything around the building such as graffiti or something that was broken I would make note of it and contact the landlord right away.

Once I got inside my office I would walk around and make sure everything looked and felt the way I wanted it to. It was important to be sure that the way my office looked was consistent with the level of excellence that we were looking to accomplish each day.

If there were chairs moved out of place I would move them back. If there were magazines or brochures on the floor or other places that I didn't want them I would sort them out properly. I would also look at the pictures on the walls to be sure they weren't tilted and if they were, I fixed them.

Another important reason for arriving early was it gave me an opportunity to pray over my practice. As I walked room by room investigating I would also pray for God's blessings on what would happen in each of those rooms on that day.

Knowing that sick and suffering people had come to my practice and were made well, I would thank God for the blessings of the previous day and remind myself of the great work He was doing there. I would also ask for His blessings on the current day.

By the time my first team member arrived I was already spiritually, emotionally, and mentally prepared for a great day.

I would assess my team members to see how their attitudes were during our short morning meeting. In that meeting, we would pray together as a team, remind ourselves of the great work we did on the previous day, and go over the schedule to get excited about what we were going to do that day.

By this point, it was about 15 minutes before we opened the doors and I would go into a quiet place and prepare my mind and body for a great day of adjusting. I would begin with stretches and exercises that would prepare my body as I thought through and visualized the great work we were going to do that day. My team would check messages and get everything prepared and ready to unlock the door.

We would unlock the door five minutes before opening time and be ready with our music playing, tea brewing, and smiles on our faces ready to greet and give our patients an awesome experience!

There is a drastic difference to this kind of intentional and purposeful morning compared to arriving five minutes before your first patient, quickly rushing in to check your schedule and walking in to adjust your first patient while you still have your keys in your pocket.

WORK ETHIC

"Working hard or hardly working" may be a silly phrase but many Upper Cervical Doctors and their teams are not really working hard every day.

Set the standard in your practice of hard work and your team will follow suit.

Make sure your team is cluster booking all of your patients if possible. If you only have 10 patients to see that day, try to see all 10 in an hour. My friend Dr. Noel Lloyd talks about having power hours where you schedule only existing patients for check and adjust or check and non-adjust appointments and no special appointments (new patients, report findings, progress exams etc.) during 2 to 3 hours per day.

Scheduling in these type of power hours each day is a tremendous way to get more efficient and feel, prepare, and train you and your team for the physical, mental, and emotional impact of truly working hard.

Those of you who are already busy and see a good patient flow know how great it feels, you may be tired at the end of the day but you probably also feel excited and accomplished.

However, if you see one patient and then go sit in your office for 20 minutes and then see a second patient and so forth, it will drain you. At the end of a day, you will feel more tired than if you saw 30 patients in three hours and you will not have the same excited feeling of accomplishment.

EFFORT

Effort goes beyond just having a good work ethic.

When you and your team put out maximum effort you will get the maximum return on your investment which will help your practice reach its full potential.

Effort is constantly thinking about how you can do things better.

When your team puts the effort in to continually innovating your processes and procedures while at the same time having a consistent work ethic you will be able to help more people, have more fun, and make more money.

Without effort, you can get stuck in a rut. You can easily get distracted from your purpose if you are not intentional with the amount of effort you're putting into all aspects of your practice.

BODY LANGUAGE

What do slumped shoulders and a frown say to your patients?

And what do a confident smile and good posture say?

A University of Michigan study revealed that 93% of all communication is body language and voice inflection.

If you and your team focus on your body language it can make a tremendous difference in how your patients feel about you and your practice.

Have you worked with your team on handshakes, eye contact, voice inflection, and body language?

Don't assume that your team knows how to handle themselves with excellence. Train yourself and your team because it can make a dramatic impact on your level of trust, credibility, and likability with your new and existing patients.

ENERGY

Is your office full of good energy?

As the clinic director, it is your responsibility to be the CEO of your practice...the Chief Energy Officer.

When you bring strong positive energy to the office with you every day, your team and your patients will reflect it.

Remember that you are there to serve.

If you're having struggles at home, you have to leave them at home.

Your patients are not responsible for being your counselor.

Nothing can kill the energy of your office faster than a grumbling and complaining Doc or team member.

Be intentional about the energy that you bring to the office and your team's energy as well.

ATTITUDE

If you and your team have a strong positive mental attitude that reflects your love for Upper Cervical and your patients, people will want to refer their friends and family to come see you.

Patients refer to Doctors that they know, like, and trust. A positive mental attitude is a great starting point for developing that "know, like and trust" factor.

Having a great attitude is a habit. It starts with knowing your purpose and being intentional about your thought patterns as we talked about in the last chapter.

Your attitude is an outward representation of your inner mindset. So the consistency of your attitude in your practice can make a tremendous difference in the attitude of your team members and your patients.

PASSION

In the last chapter, we talked about the importance of enthusiasm as a mindset of the world's top Upper Cervical Doctors. Once again we see that when you have an inner enthusiasm in your mindset you can exude passion as a habit in your work on a daily basis.

If you love what you do and are passionate about the work and the patients that you get to serve that will be reflected in every interaction of every day.

Passion is contagious.

BEING COACHABLE

I am a strong proponent of coaching. I have had coaches for my Upper Cervical Practice, my online marketing agency, fitness coaches, and even a coach for this book.

There is a reason why the most successful professional athletes in the world have coaches.

Coaching works. If you don't have a coach you should get one.

And you should also be coaching your team so that they can be more successful in your practice and in life.

My experience is consistent with the world's top Upper Cervical Doctors.

Consistently on the podcast doctors have discussed the importance of mentorship and coaching as a key ingredient in their success.

Invest in good coaching.

There are a number of excellent chiropractic coaches who work with Upper Cervical Doctors including:

- Dr. Noel Lloyd – Five Star Management
  http://www.myfivestar.com/

- Dr. Jeff Scholten – Healthy ChiroPractice
  https://www.healthychiropractice.com/
- Dr. Todd Osborne – AMC https://www.amcfamily.com/
- Dr. Justin Brown – New Beginnings Chiropractic Life Coaching
  https://chiropracticlifecoaching.com/
- Dr. Robert Brooks – Taking Care Of People
  http://www.tcopseminar.com/consulting-services.html

DOING EXTRA

It is never crowded on the extra mile.

When you go the extra mile for your team, your patients, or your family, then you will receive the greater reward.

Doing extra takes effort but its well worth it.

Whenever possible under promise and over deliver to your patients. This is one of the most effective ways to create raving fans.

BEING PREPARED

When you go in to do a report of findings for a new patient how prepared are you?

When you are prepared you are more confident. When you are prepared you will have more certainty.

Don't ever walk into a report of findings and just wing it. That person deserves better than that.

In AMC they used to talk about the hand on the door principle. The goal is that before you open any door in your office you have a mental picture of what you're looking to accomplish in that interaction. The more effectively you prepare for patient or team interactions the better the results of those interactions will be.

During this first section, we have focused on personal mastery. When you take a realistic look at your life on a regular basis, master your mindset, and consistently cultivate winning habits you are preparing yourself for practice mastery which is what we will discuss in the next section.

SECTION 2:
PRACTICE MASTERY

"Practice is the price of mastery. Whatever you practice over and over again becomes a new habit of thought and performance."

– Brian Tracy

CHAPTER FOUR

CAST YOUR PRACTICE VISION

Developing Your Practice Core Values, Mission, Vision, and Goals

*"Vision is a picture of the future that
produces passion."*

– Bill Hybels

Up to this point, we have really focused on you personally, but now it's time to get into the nuts and bolts of how to master a successful Upper Cervical Practice.

When we started the mindset chapter we talked about the importance of your purpose in establishing a winning mindset.

Likewise, the first aspect of mastering Upper Cervical Practice is taking your personal purpose and applying it within your practice to guide you in establishing your practice core values, mission, vision, and goals.

When you establish core values, vision, and mission effectively it will make an impact on everything you do in your practice.

The work that it will take to determine the things that are important to you, your team, and your patients will pay off in both the short and long term.

Also, once you have these key components in place for your practice it will be much easier to make decisions when it comes to goals that need to be set, team members that need to be hired, training that needs to be done, etc.

The most successful companies in the world focus on the importance of core values with <u>80% of the Fortune 100 touting their values publicly,</u> and there is abundant evidence that companies with a high sense of purpose <u>outperform others by 400%</u>.

So, let's take a look at each of these key components.

CORE VALUES

Core values are essentially what your company is all about.

This collection of characteristics outlines what it means to be a team member of your practice.

For instance, here are our core values at Upper Cervical Marketing:

<u>Team</u> – We are team members, not employees. This is not just a job, we are doing work that matters. Our team is on a mission to help sick and suffering people all over the world. We win together or we lose together. We reward performance and results on our team. We have fun and enjoy working together as a team.

<u>Family Matters</u> – We balance family with working hard. We give ourselves adequate time to rest and recover with our friends and family and to enjoy the fruits of our labor. We encourage the development of friendships within our team. By giving ourselves margin we are fresh and ready to do our important work that matters.

<u>Communication with Consideration</u>- Whether through email, phone, in-person or online meetings our team is considerate of each other and communicate with clarity and gratitude. We treat others the way we want to be treated and keep in mind the best interest of our team, company, clients and their potential patients. We pass negatives up and positives all around and avoid gossip at all times.

<u>Trustworthiness</u>- We believe we are in the trust business. We believe marketing is all about building trust, credibility, and likability. We value that we can trust one another on our team. That our clients can trust us as their online marketing department. And that sick and suffering patients can trust the marketing messages we design for our clients.

<u>Self-responsibility</u>- Accountability, and ownership of responsibilities are hallmarks of our team. We act like we own the company and have a self-employed mentality. As a mobile and global team, we take ownership of the clients we work for and the responsibilities we perform regardless of where we are in the world. We believe character matters all the time.

Continual Innovation- We understand the ever-changing industry with which we work and appreciate the importance of testing and iterating in order to find the best practices for every location and market. Continual innovation helps us acquire new clients and retain the clients who have trusted their marketing to us.

Excellence in the Ordinary- We believe in a standard of personal integrity where you own your successes and failures without diminishing or exaggerating your contribution to either. We believe in focusing on our specific strength areas and are faithful in the little things. We believe that diligence is excellence in the ordinary over time and through diligence, we will prosper in our mission.

These core values are the foundational pillars of our company.

We look for these characteristic values in team members we hire and we hold each other accountable to this standard.

If a team member is not living up to our core values we will call them out on it. A lack of congruence to our core values is the number one reason why someone is no longer working with our team.

The best way for you to determine what your core values should be for your practice is to first determine what is most important to you.

Go back to your purpose that we investigated in chapter 2 and really make sure you know what your purpose is and how your practice is helping you accomplish it.

Next, you're going to do a core values brainstorm.

This is how you do it.

Start thinking about words that come to mind as you go through these questions about your practice.

- What is the initial impression or feeling people have as they approach your office?
- How do people feel when they walk into your lobby?
- How do people feel when they call your practice?
- How do patients feel when they meet you for the first time?
- What is a patients' first visit like in your office?

- How do you want your patients to feel?
- What do you want the atmosphere to be like?
- How do you want your team members to feel about the company?
- If a patient was describing your practice to someone else what words would you want them to use?
- If one of your team members was describing your practice to someone else what words would you want them to use?
- If you were telling a friend about your practice how would you describe it?

Begin to capture words as you go through this brainstorm.

The more words you have the better.

Next go through and circle different words that are the most important of the ones that are written down.

It is also good to get input from your team and patients especially if they have been with you for a while about what is most important to them about the practice.

Once you have accumulated core values that are essential to you and your team you can then begin to translate those into core values that can be permeated throughout the culture of your practice.

Make sure that you are not overdoing it with values.

Shoot for 3 to 7 core values (maximum of 10)

MISSION

Next, create a one-sentence mission that your team can rally behind.

You want to make sure that it's something that you are all very passionate about.

Your mission should focus on a bigger purpose.

Our mission at Upper Cervical Marketing is:

"Our Upper Cervical Marketing Team is on a **mission to help sick and suffering people all over the world find _HOPE AND HEALING_**

through Upper Cervical Doctors in their community."

You'll notice that this mission is what starts our vision as well in the next section.

Again, focus on a statement that is a crusade for your practice.

A rallying cry that you can all get behind and say, "Yes! I do that every day".

At Upper Cervical Marketing we love giving people hope and seeing people get well which is why this mission statement is perfectly suited for us.

Over the past 5 years, we have helped over 20,000 new patients find their way to Upper Cervical Doctors throughout the world.

Make sure your mission gets you fired up and also fires your team up!

Is Your Team Passionate About Your Mission?

If you have a person on your team that is not passionate about your mission, well simply put, that is a big problem.

You have got to make sure that you have the right people on your team and get the wrong people off of your team. The right people are the ones that are fired up about your mission, vision and core values.

We will talk more about the importance of hiring the right CA'S, Office Manager, and Associates later in the book.

However, I cannot stress enough that if you hire the right people the problem of how to motivate and manage them will largely disappear. If you find that you are constantly having to manage and motivate your employee(s) then it is likely that you have made a hiring mistake.

Communicate Your Mission to Your Patients

Dr. Terry McCoskey discussed the importance of translating your mission and vision to your patients as well in one of our interviews:

"Yes, in fact, we think the people in our practice become part of our mission and vision. Our mission and vision revolve around helping people understand their responsibility and their role in managing their health. I think of it no differently than if you saw somebody drowning you would throw them a rope, so when you see somebody suffering it's your responsibility as somebody who knows the whole truth now. It's a responsibility that you have to say, "Hey, if I had something that could help you would you like me to tell you?"

Whether it's your spouse, a family member, or a friend that you see at church, or at the grocery store, maybe a complete stranger. **We coach our patients into being part of our mission and vision and to serve as many people as we can**. Yes, it's a responsibility we all have, once you know the truth you're accountable for sharing it."

In episode 16 of the Upper Cervical Marketing Podcast, Dr. Ian Davis-Tremayne discussed his practice vision and how it plays out day-to-day in his practice.

Here are some quotes from that interview:

Dr. Ian Davis-Tremayne: "...I wanted everyone to be able to afford care in whatever way they could, and so I wanted to build a clinic that you walked into and immediately when you walk into, you feel like you're in a healing path..I wanted to create that community-based feeling where people can rent out our space and they could have talks, they could have classes."

"You walk in, you feel calm, you feel collected, and you're ready to be served. We have a lot of people come in and they just like to hang in our lounge, and whether they get adjusted or checked or whatever, they still enjoy being there."

Dr. Davis-Tremayne continues "I offer a sliding scale if needed to everybody. So, they all know it's a possibility if they absolutely needed it, and if you pull up in a beautiful Tesla or a Ferrari, I still mention the sliding scale, and most people are like, 'No, no. I'm good,' and they're fine, but the other people who need it, they're really appreciative of that, and they don't get less care. They don't get less energy from me. They get care just like anybody else would."

This is his practice mission and vision, but my practice mission and vision were very different and yours will be different as well.

Remember your practice is a reflection of you so make sure that your unique practice core values, mission, and vision are consistent with who you are as a person.

VISION

Now that you know your core values and mission for your practice you will want to begin establishing your vision.

Here are some questions to ask yourself to help write your initial vision:

- What will your practice look like when it's done?
- How many patients would you like to see on a weekly basis?
- How many new patients would you like to see on a monthly basis?
- What is your target for collections each month?
- How many team members will work in the practice?
- What will your role be?

A good way to break down the vision is into 3 basic sections:

- **Who We Are**
- **Who Our Patients Are**
- **Where We Are Going**

Here is an excerpt from the "who we are" section of our Upper Cervical Marketing vision:

"Our Upper Cervical Marketing Team is on a **mission to help sick and suffering people all over the world find _HOPE AND HEALING_ through Upper Cervical Doctors in their community.**

We serve our Upper Cervical Specific Chiropractic Clients so they can serve more people in their communities with life-changing Upper Cervical Care.

We offer Digital marketing services exclusively to Upper Cervical Doctors in all English-speaking nations including the United States, Canada, Australia, New Zealand, South Africa, United Kingdom and the Philippines.

Our leadership team believes in empowering our team members. We believe that we can either have control or growth but not both. So, we delegate authority and not just tasks to develop leaders.

All of our team members are either Upper Cervical Doctors or experts in online marketing.

We are large enough to serve a large number of clients but efficient enough in our processes and systems to feel like a smaller company with personal service to our clients."

You want to keep your vision to less than 3 pages and focus on those 3 main sections.

Now that you have your values, mission, and vision in place you can make decisions and set goals that are consistent with these foundational pillars.

GOALS

Now that you have a good understanding of your practice core values, mission, and vision you can begin to set goals that are consistent with your core values and mission and will help your practice accomplish your vision.

Execution is the key when it comes to turning your vision into a reality. I discussed this in detail with Dr. Christopher Wolff in episode 42 of the podcast and it all comes down to goal setting.

Your practice should set the following goals:

- 10 Year Target (BHAG)
- 3 Year Picture
- One Year Goals
- Quarterly Priorities (12 week year)
- Monthly Key Performance Indicators

YOUR PRACTICE'S 10 YEAR TARGET (BHAG)

Your ten-year target needs to be **A BIG GOAL!**

It's what Jim Collins called in his book Built to Last a **Big Hairy Audacious Goal** (BHAG for short).

According to Collins: *"A true BHAG is clear and compelling, serves as a unifying focal point of effort...It has a clear finish line, so the organization can know when it has achieved the goal. It is tangible, energizing, highly focused. People get it right away; it takes little or no explanation."*

It is very important that you and your team have created and are pursuing a BHAG for your practice.

Without a clearly defined BIG GOAL that your team is driving towards, your results will be limited.

Examples of BHAG's include:

- Stanford University's goal in the 1940s was to become the "Harvard of the West."
- Boeing in 1950 wanted to become the "dominant player in commercial aircraft and bring the world into the jet age."
- Nike's goal in the 1960s was to "Crush Adidas."
- Wal-Mart, in 1990, wanted to become a "$125 billion company by the year 2000."

Set correctly, BHAGs work.

But how do you do that for your Upper Cervical Practice?

Taking clues from Collins and Porras, a good BHAG has four qualities:

- **Aligned.** Properly set goals can be transformational if they're tied closely to what is most important to your practice (core values, mission, and vision). The goal needs to be specific enough that everyone will know if you achieve it.
- **Audacious.** BHAGs are a breed apart. They're very, very, very big. You're probably on to something if the first reaction to a BHAG is "impossible!" BHAGs can't be achieved easily or quickly. It demands different thinking.
- **Articulate.** A good BHAG is a clear target. And it's real. It's not in any way a fanciful statement disconnected from the business. Kennedy's 1961 mission to "land on the moon by the end of the decade" needs no further detail.
- **Arduous.** Easy goals don't require innovation. A good BHAG does. It's achievable, but only through different thinking, a real struggle. When you first set your BHAG you won't yet know the details of how to accomplish the goal. However, if it's truly impossible—as opposed to perceived as impossible—people will disengage from the process entirely.

Here are some additional tips on writing this BHAG with your team:

- Jim Collins' BHAG acronym contains the word "big", but just setting some lofty growth target 5 to 10 years into the future is not necessarily going to inspire your team.
- It's really not about being "big" as much as it's about being "great", however you choose to define greatness.
- Imagine it is 10 years into the future. What great achievement, if your practice was able to accomplish it, would make you think that you spent those 10 years of your life wisely?

So now it's your turn.

Spend some time brainstorming with your team about your Big Hairy Audacious Goal!

YOUR PRACTICE'S 3 YEAR PICTURE

Your practice's 3-year picture needs to be building towards your 10-year target BHAG. It should have a specific date that it will be accomplished, it should be measurable, and should include a description of what it looks like.

Here's an example:

Future Date:
December 31st, 2021

Measurable:
200 people helped (patient visits) per week or more for 12 consecutive weeks

What Does It Look Like?
Our team of 4 (clinic director, associate, office manager, front desk assistant) is living out our core values in the service of our community.

We are consistently delivering high-quality care with maximum efficiency. 60% or more of our new patients are coming from referral.

We are consistently collecting video testimonials and online reviews from our raving fans.

ONE YEAR GOALS

Once you have established your 10-year target and your 3-year picture, next you can lay out your one-year goals.

Your one-year goals should be S.M.A.R.T. goals.

- **Specific** (simple, sensible, significant) – you can't just say I want my practice to grow this year. You need to specifically state how much growth you want.

- **Measurable** (meaningful, motivating) – the goal needs to be measurable. You need to know if you hit it or not. We are looking for specific numbers and metrics.

- **Achievable** (agreed, attainable) – if your practice collected $100,000 last year and this year your goal is to collect $1 million that is most likely not attainable. You don't want to make it so completely ridiculous when it comes to a one-year goal that your team will be demotivated.

- **Relevant** (reasonable, realistic and resourced, results-based) – This step is about ensuring that your goal matters to you and that it also aligns with other relevant goals. We all need support and assistance in achieving our goals, but it's important to retain control over them. So, make sure that your plans drive everyone forward, but that you're still responsible for achieving your own goal.

  o A relevant goal can answer "yes" to the following questions:

    ▪ Does this seem worthwhile?
    ▪ Is this the right time?
    ▪ Does this match our other efforts/needs?
    ▪ Am I the right person to reach this goal?
    ▪ Is it applicable to the current socio-economic environment?

- **Timely** (time-based, time-limited, time/cost limited, timely, time-sensitive) – the last aspect of a smart goal for your practice is to put a specific date by which it will be accomplished.

At a very minimum, you want to set goals each year about your numbers including:

- patient visits
- new patients
- collections
- overhead
- office visit average

You might also want to set other goals such as personal vacation days, team social events, patient referrals generated, profit, etc.

We will talk more about statistics later in the book.

ALIGNING YOUR TEAM'S PERSONAL GOALS WITH THE PRACTICE'S GOALS

A great tip that I got from one of our top Upper Cervical Doctors that we have interviewed over the years was from Dr. Larry Arbeitman.

Dr. Arbeitman makes a point to understand all of his team members personal goals whether it be vacations they want to take, getting their child into private school, or running a marathon.

He then shows his team members how if the practice accomplishes certain goals it will allow the team member to also accomplish their personal goal.

Intrinsic motivation will always be powerful and the more effectively you can align your practice goals with the personal goals of your team, the more likely you are to accomplish them together.

Dr. Jeff Scholten also discussed this in episode one of the Upper Cervical Marketing Podcast.

Here is a paraphrased quote from our interview:

Dr. Scholten: "…you have to be on the same page. It's so important…I remember, a couple of years into practice, I went to a NUCCA conference (and the following week) was the busiest week we'd ever had (in practice). It was Friday…and we were having our end of the day meeting. (I asked my staff) "How's next week looking?"

46

One of my two team members at that time said, 'Oh, it's better next week.' I said, 'what do you mean? How can it be better? She said 'well, it's not as busy.' And, I realized at that point… the busier I was, it really increased my profit margin.

Dr. Scholten continued: **But for her, at her hourly wage, the busier she was, decreased her dollar per energy expenditure. So, we had to switch that. What we do now is we have four bonus levels that we give out on a monthly basis, based on how that month was. We understand that there's a certain percentage number of our revenue at the end of the day that should go to our employees. We try to make sure that (the profit sharing) encourages them. So, they know if they're busy working the phones hard and they're moving people around and they're running, running, running that they're actually getting paid more per minute than if they're just sitting there playing solitaire.**

So, that's the key to get these procedures in place so that everything is lining up. So, whether it's your patients or your team, **we all have to be moving towards the same end goal**." Said Dr. Scholten.

QUARTERLY PRIORITIES AND THE 12 WEEK YEAR

Now that you have your one-year goals you can establish your quarterly priorities (**12-week goals**) or what Stephen Covey calls "your rocks".

12-week goals are the bridge between your vision and your action plan.

Your action plans prioritize your work on a daily and weekly basis.

These are the 1-3 extra projects above and beyond your daily work that each team member is going to accomplish in this particular quarter to move you towards your long term goals and targets. These priorities should be checked in on every week during your team meeting (which we will talk about later in the book) to make sure each team member is making progress towards the completion of their priorities.

This is the time when having a solid execution system in place becomes critical. In the book, the 12 Week Year: Get More Done in 12 Weeks Than Others Do in 12 Months by Brian Moran and Michael Lennington, the authors lay out an extremely effective execution system that I use personally and in our business.

Here's how it works.

- It starts with all the steps we have already discussed. Creating your core values, mission, vision, 10-year target, 3-year picture and one-year goals.
- Then have each team member pick **one goal** that they want to accomplish over the next 12 weeks that will help the practice move closer to your one year, 3 year, 10-year goals, and vision. I also do this with personal goals. I like to have 1-3 12-week professional goals and 1-3 12 week personal goals each quarter.
- Think through all of the actions that need to take place to accomplish the 12-week goal. Some of these need to be done once and others every week or over several weeks.
- Now list which week each action needs to be completed in order to accomplish the goal.
- Next layout the entire 12-week plan with all of the actions and the weeks they need to be completed.
- For week one print out the actions you need to take that week and do them. Continue for week two, week three and so forth.
- At the end of each week during your weekly meeting with your team, keep track of the actions completed the previous week and give yourself a score out of 100%. Such as if you had 4 actions to complete and you only completed 2 then your score would be 50%. You want to maintain at least an 85% average at completing your action items in order to ensure you will accomplish your 12-week goal.

The 12 Week Year book has a companion software that I use and really like to help track your actions, score your execution, and accomplish better results. You can get it at https://12weekyear.com/achieve/.

After 12 weeks (during the 13th week – the last week of the quarter), ask yourself how your situation has changed and what new opportunities have presented themselves, and create new 12-week goals.

MONTHLY KEY PERFORMANCE INDICATORS

The last set of goals that top practices have are monthly Key Performance Indicators (KPIs). A KPI is a metric that is associated with a specific result.

Each team member should have clearly identified expected results called

Key Results Areas (KRA's) with specific and measurable numbers associated with them (KPIs).

These metrics should be reviewed during your weekly team meetings to make sure everyone is on target to hit your KPI's for that month. We will talk more about KRA's and KPIs later in the book.

Laying out your core values, vision, mission, and goals will get you one step closer to Upper Cervical Practice Mastery.

To take a deeper dive into the principles laid out in this chapter and the entire book go to http://uppercervicalpracticemastery.com/academy to learn more about the companion course that goes along with this *Upper Cervical Practice Mastery* book. The companion course contains worksheets, tools, in-depth webinars about each chapter, email Q&A, and exclusive access to a private Facebook group for accountability and community with other doctors and students looking to become Upper Cervical Practice Masters.

CHAPTER FIVE

MASTER YOUR UPPER CERVICAL TECHNIQUE

You Have Got To Deliver the Goods

"We are all apprentices in a craft where no one ever becomes a master."

– Ernest Hemingway

Now that you have worked on your personal mastery and have laid out your core values, vision, mission, and goals the next step is making sure that you are on a journey to mastering your Upper Cervical Technique.

You can never completely master any of the Upper Cervical Techniques and if you think you have I guarantee that there is always something more to learn.

But if you can't deliver the goods, then what's the point?

On the flipside, you could be the greatest technician in the world but if you do not master the other aspects of Upper Cervical Practice as discussed in this book, you will very likely fail.

There are many Upper Cervical Doctors that were incredibly skilled adjusters and now they are doing construction, teaching at a college, selling real estate, or something else besides Upper Cervical because their practice was not successful.

Therefore, it is imperative that you make sure you are mastering ALL aspects of Upper Cervical Practice.

INVEST IN YOUR TECHNIQUE

You owe it to your community to be the best possible Upper Cervical Chiropractic analyzer and adjuster that you can be.

Your patient's results are the fuel that drives everything else.

If you're getting great results and changing lives on a daily basis it will fuel your passion.

It will fuel your team's passion.

It will drive your patients to want to refer others.

We are going to teach you later in the book how you can harness your success stories to spread the word in your community about what is happening in your office. This excitement will help to fuel your entire community's health improvement.

Once you have determined which Upper Cervical Technique resonates with you best, pursue it to the highest level of certification. Continue to go to seminars every year. Don't ever think that you've arrived or that you know enough. It's crucial that you are keeping your skills fresh through accountability with your colleagues. Getting together to regularly practice the fundamentals of your analyzing and adjusting technique will help to ensure you are providing the best care possible for your patients.

UPPER CERVICAL DIPLOMATE

In addition, to seeking certification and ongoing learning within your chosen Upper Cervical Technique, I would also highly recommend the Upper Cervical Diplomate Program through the ICA's Council on Upper Cervical Care.

The diplomate gives you an in-depth understanding of the anatomy, neurology, and physiology of the Upper Cervical Spine and its impact on the brain and the body. It will also give you an understanding of the most widely used Upper Cervical Approaches as well as more well-rounded and in-depth ways to help you care for difficult cases.

The Upper Cervical Diplomate Program focuses on advanced imaging techniques including upright MRI, CBCT and other advanced imaging. These techniques are becoming more and more important in today's world and are an excellent way to start conversations with the medical community.

You can find more information about the diplomate program here http://www.icauppercervical.com/Diplomate-Program.

BIG PICTURE THINKING

Another characteristic I have found from interviewing top Upper Cervical Doctors is their focus on big-picture thinking.

The top doctors in our profession tend to think about the big picture and tend to focus on how to support and grow Upper Cervical as a whole.

They avoid isolationism and invest both monetarily and in a voluntary capacity to their Upper Cervical Technique and other chiropractic organizations for the betterment of the profession.

You will find that many of the most successful upper cervical doctors are also some of the most involved doctors within our profession. Doctors like Dr. Jeff Scholten, Dr. Julie Mayer-Hunt, and Dr. Kerry Johnson are very involved with their technique organizations as well as other Upper Cervical focused organizations to advance research and Upper Cervical both politically and educationally.

It would be beneficial for you to get involved with the leadership of your technique organization and also with the ICA Council on Upper Cervical Care http://www.icauppercervical.com/Join-Us to help advance Upper Cervical worldwide.

THE TECHNICIAN, THE MANAGER, AND THE ENTREPRENEUR

In this chapter, we have really focused on you as a technician.

In Michael Gerber's fantastic book, *The E Myth Revisited*, he discusses the importance of a successful small business owner being a technician, a manager, and an entrepreneur.

In the chapters to follow, we will continue to investigate and learn how to be an effective manager and entrepreneur so that your technical skills can serve your community effectively.

CHAPTER SIX

SUCCEED WITH YOUR TEAM

Hire and Develop Team Members to Accomplish Your Goals

"Great things in business are never done by one person. They're done by a team of people."

– Steve Jobs

Your team can either be your greatest asset or your greatest downfall.

In about 90% of the cases, the first person someone speaks to in your practice is not you.

Have you really thought about that?

In the large majority of cases, the first impression of the practice is not made by you. The initial phone conversation with your practice can make or break you.

Do you have any idea how many new patients you lose because of these conversations?

If you have not hired the right people for your team or have not consistently invested in training, then it is likely that you are losing many new patients based solely on these phone conversations.

It's important that you confront this reality so you can do something about it.

The first step is hiring team members who are consistent with your core values.

HIRING IDEAL TEAM PLAYERS

When it comes to hiring, a fantastic book to read is the *Ideal Team Player by Patrick Lencioni*. In his book, Lencioni describes the 3 characteristics of an Ideal Team Player for any organization:

- Humble
- Hungry
- Smart

HUMBLE

As we talked about in chapter 2 one of the key characteristics of a top Upper Cervical Doctor's mindset is humility and you likewise want to look for a similar mindset in the team members that you hire.

During the hiring process get the potential team member to talk about their past work and projects. Listen closely to the words that they use.

Are they very **I** focused in their descriptions or very **we** focused?

Humble people tend to talk more about what the team was able to accomplish rather than what they were able to do themselves.

You can also ask them to discuss their weaknesses. Humble people understand that they have strengths and weaknesses and are not afraid to admit that.

Humble people are quick to point out the contributions of others and slow to seek attention for their own.

They lack excessive ego or concerns about status.

They share credit, emphasize team over self and define success collectively rather than individually.

This is the kind of person that you want on your team regardless of your core values.

HUNGRY

Along with humility, an ideal team player is hungry.

As Jim Collins described the Level V Leadership characteristics of the Good to Great companies in his book you are looking for someone that has a **personal humility and a professional ambition**.

There focus is on the patient and the team and not on themselves.

Ask them during the interview to talk about a time when they needed to go above and beyond and put in extra hours in order to accomplish a goal either personally or professionally.

They are always looking for more.

More things to do.

More to learn.

More responsibility to take on.

Hungry people almost never have to be pushed by a manager to work harder because they are self-motivated and diligent.

They are constantly thinking about the next step and the next opportunity.

SMART

Lastly, an ideal team player is smart.

Not just that they have intelligence, but they are people smart. They understand how to communicate with people and have a solid relational intelligence.

They have common sense about people.

Smart people tend to know what is happening in a group situation and how to deal with others in the most effective way.

They have good judgment and intuition around the subtleties of group dynamics and the impact of their words and actions.

I recommend doing group interviews. When you have 10 to 15 candidates in your lobby, watch how they interact with each other and with your current team members.

Also, during the interview how does the person make you feel?

Someone that is people smart will be good with people and will be able to communicate in a way that makes you feel comfortable. We have a basic assessment to assess these three virtues in the companion course for this book.

Learn more and get access at
http://uppercervicalpracticemastery.com/academy

UNDERSTANDING PERSONALITIES AND STRENGTHS

Along with the ideal team player virtues, the top Upper Cervical Doctors also understand the personalities and strengths of their potential team members to see if they're the right fit for the position that they're looking to hire.

There are a variety of different personality evaluations that you can use during the hiring process including:

- DISC
- Enneagram
- Strength Finders

Each of these have their strengths and weaknesses but the one that I have personally found the most value from is the DISC profile.

DISC is an acronym that stands for the four main personality types of all human beings.

D = Driver (dominating, determined, direct, demanding)

People with the D style personality are task driven and place an emphasis on shaping the environment by overcoming opposition to accomplish results.

A person with a D style personality:

- Is motivated by winning, competition and success.
- Prioritizes accepting a challenge, taking action and achieving immediate results.

- Is described as direct, demanding, forceful, strong-willed, driven, determined, fast-paced, and self-confident.

I = Influencer (interactive, impulsive, influential)

People with the I style personality are people focused and place an emphasis on shaping the environment by influencing or persuading others.

A person with an I style personality:

- May be limited by being impulsive, disorganized and having lack of follow-through
- Are described as convincing, magnetic, enthusiastic, warm, trusting and optimistic
- Prioritizes taking action, collaboration, and expresses enthusiasm
- Is motivated by social recognition, group activities, and relationships

S = Steady (secure, sensitive, supportive, stable)

People with the S style personality are people oriented and place an emphasis on cooperating with others within existing circumstances to carry out the task.

A person with an S style personality:

- Is motivated by cooperation, opportunities to help and sincere appreciation
- Prioritizes giving support, collaboration and maintaining stability
- Is described as calm, patient, predictable, deliberate, stable and consistent.
- May be limited by being indecisive, overly accommodating and tendency to avoid change
- May fear change, loss of stability and offending others.
- Values loyalty, helping others and security

C = Conscientious (consistent, analytical, calculating, cautious)

People with the C style personality are task oriented and place an emphasis on working conscientiously within existing circumstances to ensure quality and accuracy.

A person with a C style personality:

- Is motivated by opportunities to gain knowledge, show their expertise, and do quality work.
- Prioritizes accuracy, stability, and challenging assumptions.
- Is described as careful, cautious, systematic, diplomatic, accurate and tactful.
- May be limited by being overcritical, overanalyzing, and isolating themselves.
- Values quality and accuracy

The first step in understanding personalities is understanding yourself.

If you don't know where you stand with the DISC profile I recommend you take the test yourself and get the full assessment.

You can get it from a variety of places but my company uses the assessment you can purchase from Dave Ramsey here since it has all the test and excellent explanations of how to use it effectively in your business https://www.daveramsey.com/store/budgeting-tools/online-tools/disc-assessment-test/proddisc.html or just search "Dave Ramsey DISC profile".

Once you understand your personality type next you can begin looking for different personalities for different roles within your company.

If you are a High D or High C and you have only one team member, then I would recommend you hire either a High S or a High I. High D or High C is very task oriented and can struggle to connect with people at times. This is where a High S or High I who is very people oriented can really help balance out the office.

The opposite would be true if you are a High I or High S then it would be ideal for you to have a High D or High C to help you stay on task.

In my office, I went through six CA's in my first six months!

It was a nightmare. I made every mistake possible and when I finally found a solid front desk person who later became my office manager she was humble, hungry, and smart but she also had a complementary personality to mine that made our practice really come alive.

If you have multiple team members a variety of personalities can really help the team work well together.

Currently, on our team at Upper Cervical Marketing, we have 16 team members and we have all four of the personality profile types represented.

It's important that everyone on the team honors the diversity of the team and that all team members are grateful for the skills and abilities their fellow team members bring to the table. Once again we have a basic assessment to assess these DISC Profile in the companion course for this book. Learn more and get access at http://uppercervicalpracticemastery.com/academy

Once you pick your team members based on how humble, hungry, and smart they are and their unique personality type, the next step is to set clear expectations with a position agreement that defines the outcomes and metrics you expect clearly.

POSITION AGREEMENTS, KRA'S, AND KPI'S

A Position Agreement is an agreement between you and a team member about what the position is all about.

To be unclear is to be unkind.

The goal of the position agreement is to clearly lay out the responsibilities of the position and what success looks like.

The position agreement should include:

- Key Result Areas
- Key Performance Indicators
- Company Core Values
- Company Standards
- Signature Section

The position agreement should include the key results areas for the position and the key performance indicators which we will discuss below.

The position agreement should also include your company core values and any standards that you expect all team members to follow. There should also be a section for signatures for both you and your team member.

Key Result Area(s) (KRA'S)

A KRA is the outcome or results that you're looking for the team member to accomplish in their position on a daily basis.

A good KRA includes the ongoing responsibilities of the position and the purpose and benefits of performing those responsibilities.

Tasks and activities that focus on one or more specific area are grouped together.

Whatever is expected must be in writing, reviewed, agreed upon, and signed by both the team member and the leader so there's no confusion when something isn't getting done.

Example:

Front Desk CA KRA's

1. Create a positive first impression with new patients on the phone and in the office
2. Efficiently and effectively process patients through the office flow
3. Generate referrals from existing and new patients

For each KRA the team member should have at least one KPI to measure success.

Key Performance Indicator(s) (KPI'S)

A KPI is a quantifiable metric or measurement used to evaluate the success of a team member or team, in meeting objectives for performance associated with a KRA.

These are the metrics that matter for each team member.

Examples:

Front Desk CA KPI's: new patients scheduled, patients processed, referrals generated etc.

Office Manager KPI's: money collected, referrals generated etc.

Associate KPI'S: new patients generated, patient visits, referrals, etc.

These KPIs can be measured daily, weekly, monthly, quarterly and yearly.

We have position agreement examples with KRA's an KPI's and biannual review assessments in the companion course for this book.

Learn more and get access at
http://uppercervicalpracticemastery.com/academy

When you set clear expectations with a solid position agreement that includes KRA's and KPIs you will get much better results from your team members and they will have a much higher satisfaction in their position.

INVESTING IN YOUR TEAM DEVELOPMENT

After you hire your team members and give them clear expectations through a position agreement with KRA's and KPIs the next step is to consistently train and develop your team.

A good leader makes a team member better in their work.

A great leader makes a team member better in their life.

I spoke about this topic with Dr. Jamie Cramer on episode 26 of the podcast and she discussed the importance of weekly training and role-playing on important procedures and processes within her practice.

Most of the top Upper Cervical Doctors will do between one and three hours of training every week with their team. Each week they will pick a topic or some will have a rotating schedule of topics that they consistently train over. This would include:

- phone skills
- meeting and greeting a new patient
- consultations
- exams
- x-ray procedures
- report of findings
- financial consultations
- existing patient interactions
- progress exams

- unhappy patients
- handling objections from new patients on the phone
- gathering reviews and video testimonials

Make sure you are investing in your team with consistent training because it has a huge return on investment.

DELEGATE AND ELEVATE

Delegation is another fantastic way to develop and train team members.

There are many reasons why you may be reluctant to delegate. Many doctors struggle with the belief that only they can do _____.

The blank could be exams, x-rays, consultations, analysis, adjustments, report of findings etc.

But the truth is…

> *"You can have control or you can have growth but you can't have both."*
> **-Craig Groeschel**

In order to grow, you must give up some control and also understand that nearly every part of your business can be delegated to someone else. A common reason for your practice not continuing to grow is the fact that you are trying to wear too many hats.

You are seeing all the patients, you are taking all the x-rays, you are managing your staff, you are running your staff meetings, you are doing your bookkeeping, you are doing all of your marketing, you are doing all the talks, you are doing all the screenings, you are posting to Facebook, you are training your staff, you are casting vision for your practice, you are helping patients leave you online reviews, and on and on and on….it's exhausting! With all of that to do no wonder your practice doesn't grow. You don't have the mindset to allow for growth. There is no margin in your practice or your life.

Dr. Tom Owen used to call it the uncle principle. Where you have so much to do that you're crying "uncle" mentally which is not allowing you to grow your practice.

Your capacity is maxed out!

This also completely limits or eliminates your ability to take a vacation.

HOW TO OUTSOURCE AND DELEGATE TO GROW YOUR UPPER CERVICAL PRACTICE

When deciding what to delegate start by asking yourself these 3 questions:

- What are my top five value-producing activities in my practice?
- How do I bring the most value to my practice?
- What can I do that no one else can do?

Some answers might include:

1. Strategy
2. Vision Casting
3. Team Member Development
4. Team Training
5. Adjusting Patients (if solo practitioner)

Once you figure out your top 5 value-producing activities next you want to establish **a stop doing list**.

A stop doing list is a list of things that you want to either immediately or with time stop doing.

Here are some possible activities you may want to include on your stop doing list:

- adjusting patients
- doing consultations
- doing exams
- taking x-rays
- doing a report of findings
- gathering video testimonials and promoting them
- doing re-exams
- talking to patients about finances
- leading staff meetings
- search engine optimizing your website

- doing bookkeeping
- creating Facebook ads
- managing the schedule
- doing a patient orientation class
- doing screenings
- updating your website with new content and testimonials
- meeting with other health professionals
- submitting your website to online directories
- casting vision and communicating it to your team
- creating and modifying systems
- creating email follow-up sequences
- creating and modifying a marketing plan
- creating and promoting videos
- budgeting
- addressing patient issues
- educating patients about their health
- posting to social media
- filing
- preparing for talks
- doing reminder calls
- executing an online review strategy
- doing community talks
- training your team
- creating a monthly email newsletter
- writing checks
- executing a referral strategy
- creating landing pages
- payroll
- doing the referral paperwork when referring patients to other health professionals

And there are many other tasks that need to be completed by you or someone else every month in your practice.

Once you have your list the next step is to put the list in 3 categories:

1. Do
2. Delegate
3. Outsource

Focus on the areas that you bring the most value to as the ones that you should do. Focus on the ones that require additional training or expertise to outsource and delegate the rest to your existing team members or future team members that you will hire. A "delegate and elevate" philosophy can help take your practice to a whole different level.

When you delegate responsibility to others on your team it elevates them to a different level and also elevates you in your ability to take on the more important responsibilities for the practice and your personal life.

ASSOCIATE DEVELOPMENT

The most successful doctors in our profession have one thing in common and that is that they have a successful associate program in place.

If you do not currently have an associate(s) I want to encourage you to make this one of your goals. This is key to having the freedom, stability, and flexibility of the top Upper Cervical Doctors in our profession.

In order to have an associate(s) in your practice, your practice should be collecting at least 30,000 to 40,000 per month.

If you are not at that level yet, focus on applying the principles in this book and you will get there and then learn everything you can about developing associates effectively to go from $40,000 per month to $50,000, $60,000, $70,000 or more. Once you know how to develop associates effectively you can add additional associates to your practice systems. Featured within this book are doctors who collect 100,000, 150,000, even $200,000 per month with multiple associates.

If you can learn this crucial aspect of having a successful practice, then the sky is the limit.

But the problem, as Dr. Noel Lloyd of Five-Star Management says is...

"85% of associate relationships end poorly"

This is a major reason why many doctors avoid associate relationships. But there are many doctors who can do it successfully and I'm going to share with you some of the keys that I've learned from top Upper Cervical Doctors and consultants.

Hiring an Associate

Much of what we already went over in the team member hiring section directly applies to hiring an associate including looking for an associate that is hungry, humble, and smart. You also want to utilize the DISC assessment that we talked about earlier and make sure that their personality meshes with you and the rest of your team.

Setting Expectations

As we talked about with other team members the first step is setting clear expectations.

Once again you can do this with a solid position agreement that lays out the KRA's and KPI's of the associate position.

If you clearly communicate the outcomes that you expect as well as the metrics that you are going to use to measure those outcomes, you have a very good chance of successfully hiring an associate.

This will also help you develop a positive relationship with your associate and even if they eventually decide to move on and open their own practice, you will be much more likely to part ways on good terms.

Training and Meetings

It is extremely important to consistently train with your associate(s). At least one hour per week of role-playing and technique training is necessary. You also want to have your associate(s) in your weekly team meetings and be doing weekly one-on-one meetings with each associate.

I think the main reason that so many people have associate relationships that fail is they are not handling their team well in general and this just plays out on a larger scale with an associate who is likely your highest paid employee.

If you focus on setting clear expectations, equipping your associate for success, and holding them accountable for results, then you could develop a great associate program in your practice.

CHAPTER SEVEN

RUN YOUR UPPER CERVICAL BUSINESS

Mastering Meetings, Numbers, and Systems to Grow and Scale Your Practice

"Systems run the business and people run the systems."

– Michael Gerber

Much of what is contained in this chapter is the difference between having a good practice and a great practice.

Great practices will have great meetings, will know and interpret their numbers, and will have systems in place to scale and consistently reproduce great experiences for their patients.

MEETINGS

You must learn to love meetings.

Most meetings that happen in Upper Cervical Practices are unproductive.

But the right meetings with the right purpose can be a tremendous asset to your practice.

Along with the weekly training meetings, which we discussed in the last chapter, there are several other meetings that top Upper Cervical Doctors implement with their teams including:

- Morning Meetings
- Weekly All Team Meeting
- Weekly One-On-One Meetings
- Quarterly Planning Meetings
- Annual Planning Meeting

Morning Meetings

In the preparation section of chapter 3, I discussed the importance of preparing for your day and part of that preparation was having a morning meeting with your team.

This 10 to 15-minute meeting is a key part of having a successful day.

During this meeting you want to:

- remind yourselves of your mission
- celebrate your wins
- prepare for the day ahead

The first part of the morning meeting is just to remind your team of their mission. You can do this by simply reading your mission or you can read your mission, core values, and vision or you might choose to read different aspects of your mission, values, and vision on different days. The most important thing is to remind your team of why you do what you do.

The second part of the morning meeting is to celebrate your wins from the day before. This is when you talk about patient success stories, referrals, and other fun things that happened the day before.

The last part of the morning meeting is to look at the schedule together and prepare for the day ahead.

Do you see any bottlenecks in the schedule?

If so, see if you can call this person or that person to see if they can come 15 minutes earlier or later.

Do you see a good opening for a new patient?

If so, see if you can fill that today. The goal for this part of the meeting is to prepare your team for what lies ahead and get them excited about the lives you all are going to impact that day.

Weekly All Team Meetings

Most team meetings are unfortunately worthless, but if you are able to conduct solid meetings on a weekly basis it will greatly improve the effectiveness of your practice. One of the best books that I found on the topic of meetings and a variety of other topics as well is *Traction* by Gino Wickman. In the book, he discusses how most meetings are a 2 or 3 on a scale of 1-10, but your goal should be to have a Level 10 Meeting every week. I would recommend doing your weekly team meetings on Mondays or Tuesdays if possible.

<u>Here is a great format for a 60-minute weekly team meeting</u>:

Wins from the Week – have every team member bring one win from their week to share. This could be a patient testimonial, a personal victory, or some great progress in a project. (5 minutes)

Scorecard Review – have 5 to 6 metrics that you look at from your practice statistics from the previous week. This should include your collections, new patients, patient visits, signed care plans (or patients who started care), case fee and OVA. (5 minutes)

Quarterly Priorities – this is when each team member gives an update on their progress with their quarterly priorities or 12-week goals. These quarterly priorities (or rocks) are 1 to 3 "extra" projects that each team member is working on for that particular quarter that will help the company as a whole accomplish their one-year goals. (5 minutes)

Patient or Team Member Headlines – this could include anything that is remarkable about your patients or team members. "Mrs. Jones had her baby" ... Let's send some flowers or "my husband and I are going to Hawaii for our vacation next year". (5 minutes)

Issues – the issues section of your weekly team meetings are the most important part of the meeting. This is not just the time to grumble and complain but instead, this is the time to identify the issues that the practice is currently facing, discuss those issues, and work to resolve those issues. Every team member should have at least one issue that they have identified throughout the week. In preparation for the meeting, every team member should bring one win and one issue. For every issue, you should capture at least one to do item that is the next action towards a resolution. (25 minutes)

To Do List – as you have gone through the meeting up to this point you should have been capturing to do items. These to-do items should be assigned to a specific person or persons and be completed before the next weekly meeting. To do items could be associated with issues, headlines, priorities, scorecard or even wins. (5 minutes)

Recap to Do – the next part of the meeting is to recap the *to-do* items and pass on any messages to team members absent from the meeting. It might sound something like this: "Mary is going to call the table company to see when the part we are waiting for will arrive. Joan is going to call Mr. Jones to schedule him for a video testimonial. Dr. Davis is going to look at locations for the upcoming dinner talk." (5 minutes)

Rate the Meeting – the last part of the meeting is an opportunity to determine whether or not you had a good meeting. It's a fun and subjective way to rate the meeting and make sure that your meetings are continuing to improve. Everyone rates the meeting on a scale of 1 to 10 and you average it out and write it down on the agenda. (5 minutes)

I would recommend laying out this agenda in a spreadsheet, then go item by item and have someone keep track of time so you don't get off track.

The more you hold these meetings the easier it will be to keep the flow of the meeting and stick to your time guidelines.

Weekly One-On-One Meetings

In addition to your weekly all team meeting, I would also recommend doing a one-on-one meeting with each of your team members.

This is a 30-minute meeting that breaks down like this:

- First 10 Minutes - for them
- Second 10 Minutes – for you
- Third 10 Minutes – for development

During the first 10 minutes, they have the opportunity to talk to you about anything they want. They might tell you about a struggle they're having with a particular patient or team member. They might tell you about something that's happening in their personal life. Whatever they want to talk about during that first 10 minutes it is completely and totally up to them. I recommend asking a question like "how can I best help you today" and then just letting them talk. Take notes and really listen to what they choose to talk about.

During the second 10 minutes, this is your chance to talk to them about anything that you want. Maybe there was a particular issue that you saw and wanted to discuss with them or maybe you have a specific question to ask them. This is your opportunity to discuss anything that you need to talk with that particular team member about. Perhaps you might even need to talk a little more about what they discussed during their 10 minutes. The 10 minutes are just a guideline to drive the meeting in the direction that will be the most productive.

Some questions to ask during this portion of the meeting include:

- What have you accomplished since our last meeting?
- What are some of the hurdles that you are facing right now?
- What are you going to accomplish before our next meeting?
- How are you doing personally?

The last 10 minutes is the time to talk about the personal and professional development of the team member. I recommend having your team members read books. Leaders are readers. Within your practice, you want to cultivate leaders who are taking self-responsibility for their results within the company. Consistently encouraging team members to read good books will help them tremendously in their development. You can have them read any book that you think is important but you may want to particularly focus on those areas that you would like to see them grow. I would also recommend reading the books with them so that you can have a better discussion during this 10 minutes. If each of you read the same chapter of a great business, spiritual, or personal development book and then talk about it during this 10 minutes it will be extremely beneficial for both of you.

Annual Strategic Planning Meetings

The focus of the annual planning meeting is to lay out the things you want to accomplish the next year. This is typically done sometime between September and November. Some goals for this meeting are:

- set one-year goals
- brainstorm projects and priorities to complete during the year
- evaluate if you need to add to your team
- evaluate if you need to purchase new equipment
- evaluate if you need more space/move the office
- evaluate if you need to reorganize or redecorate
- put together a marketing calendar

This is typically a 2 to 8-hour meeting with everyone on your team.

Quarterly Planning Meetings

Once you do your annual planning meetings you then have a direction for your quarterly planning meetings. Your quarterly planning meetings should be done in the month before the quarter begins. So, a Q1 quarterly planning meeting would be done in December, Q2 would be done in March, a Q3 would be done in June and a Q4 would be done in September.

The focus of the quarterly planning meetings is to plan that particular quarter using the 12-week year execution system. You take your marketing calendar and lay out everything that you need to do in order to accomplish your marketing initiatives. You will lay out the quarterly priorities that each team member will complete for that particular quarter. You will also want to discuss any projects that need to be completed for that quarter. The more effective you are in planning the smoother your quarters will go. This meeting is typically about 2 to 4 hours.

We have a Level 10 Meeting Agenda, a One-On-One Meeting agenda, a Quarterly Planning Meeting Agenda and an Annual Strategic Planning Meeting Agenda in the companion course for this book. Learn more and get access at http://uppercervicalpracticemastery.com/academy

DEVELOPING SYSTEMS

The goal of system development is to develop systems so good that you could leave for a month and your practice would keep running and growing without you.

This means having solid systems throughout your practice including:

- phone procedures
- new patient procedures
- consultations
- examinations
- x-ray: taking and analysis
- report of findings
- daily visits
- progress exams
- healthcare classes
- financials
- CA and associate training

One of the top doctors out there when it comes to systems is Dr. Michael Lenarz. Dr. Lenarz has opened 7 Upper Cervical Chiropractic Clinics with multiple associates and we spoke in depth about systems in episode 20 of the podcast here are some paraphrased quotes.

Dr. Lenarz: "So, there's a couple of things that I think are important about systems, but I want to step back from that and see how that really fits into the broader framework of what we're doing. I think that anybody who's an Upper Cervical Doctor understands systems from a clinical perspective. The work that we have historically done in our practice is Blair work. I've worked with a lot of NUCCA doctors, AO doctors, and Orthospinology doctors. How you do the Upper Cervical Technique that you do, your systems, your procedures? How do you position the patient? How do you assess whether they need to be adjusted or whether they don't need to be adjusted? Those are all systems. Systems are very much embedded in our life."

Dr. Lenarz continues: "There are clinical systems and there are communication systems. When a doctor is generating a successful clinical outcome, it has to do with how good they are at what they do clinically and their communication techniques. How good are they at explaining things to patients and generating a relationship with patients?"

"I've got all of these systems in place to run my practices and to work with doctors but here's the thing that I realized. I never want to be on automatic. I want to be super present. Each time that I'm with the patient, I don't want to go into automatic and just do my reading, do my tests, do the adjustment, don't do the adjustment. I want to connect with the patient. I want to make sure that I'm not missing anything. I want to be present, that's how I want to live my life." Dr. Lenarz said.

"I know that in our office as an example, we have a checklist. This is part of our systems, and on that checklist, there's a whole column with 35 things on it that the front desk, the CAs or the accounts area needs to make sure gets done. On the other side of the paper is a column of things that need to be done from a clinical perspective, such as:

- have the x-rays been taken
- have the measurements been taken on the x-rays
- have we done the proper exam work
- have we prepared well for going over the information with the patient

A lot of work that goes into generating a relationship with that patient on their first, second and third visit is done to set up the foundation for that relationship. So, again for us, we have systems." Dr. Lenarz said.

"Someone comes into the office; the front desk CA knows what they're supposed to do:

- give them a tour of the office before any paperwork is done
- offer them coffee or tea or water
- have them fill out the paperwork

All of this is according to the checklist. All of this is according to training. So, we take what could possibly be somewhat haphazard and a complex amount of effort and we have systematized it and that reduces the stress level. It makes it a much more pleasant experience for the patient, the practice member, the CA, and for the doctor. It all happens smoothly." Dr. Lenarz said.

Dr. Lenarz continues "Another aspect to that is, we have systems which are communication systems including scripts:

- Scripting for day one, two and three.
- Scripting that we call a pre-consultation statement. That's when the doctor first sits down with a practice member. What do we say, how do we explain upper cervical to them?
- Scripting when we take the patient into x-ray, to be able to explain clearly what we're doing and why we're doing it.
- Scripting that we use while we are doing x-rays.
- Scripting for day two, when the patient comes back and we go through the report of findings.

Now, here's the thing about scripting. We don't really want to have everything so tightly packaged that it doesn't allow for the personal expression of the doctor. Learn good scripting on the front end and learn things that have been developed either by your coach or by other doctors who have developed these communication systems. Once you get the basics down, over time you can make that script your own."

"I'll give another example, built into the scripting is a system of education. So, oftentimes what we want to do is take a patient from a symptom-treatment paradigm to a chiropractic-philosophical paradigm. This is how we generate referrals.

The way we generate long-term lifetime care is to really get the patient to clearly understand why we do what we do, and to move from the old medical paradigm to a newer chiropractic paradigm, and the scripting that we have on day one, two and three, and the procedures that we have are also part of an underlying system of patient education to help bring the patient to this new understanding." Dr. Lenarz said.

Dr. Lenarz continues "For instance, we have a day three script, which we call retracing where we talk about retracing with the patient and explain how we don't make decisions based on symptoms. We have common communication pieces that we touch base with them on over the first few weeks that are part of that education and retention system. At six weeks in our practices, we do a re-exam. That's part of the retention system.

At 12 weeks we do another exam that's part of the retention system. So, there's another underlying system, which is geared towards retention. All of these systems are tied together. The education system, retention system, front-desk system, and clinical systems need to be streamlined to be most effective.

One of the things I've learned with patients over the last 28 years is there's not a single patient who's a textbook patient. Everybody is unique. Every situation is unique but once you get the systems down, then if you have to step outside of the system to handle a unique situation, then you can step back into the system, and it allows for the smooth operation of the business.

Even if you haven't learned any formal scripting you will generate your own scripting naturally as you consistently talk with patients about the same things. But you have to learn how to adapt to the unique situation of every single patient, and every single interaction. The scripts just help you learn how to do it well and then you can do variations on the theme."

Systems shouldn't make you robotic. Systems should free you up to be yourself in the best possible way with that individual patient.

KNOW YOUR NUMBERS:
PRACTICE STATISTICS

I once was speaking to a doctor and I asked him about some of his basic practice statistics and he said to me…

"I don't know those numbers. I know a lot of people keep numbers like that but I don't care about those numbers I just want to take care of patients."

Within a year that Doctor had closed his practice.

If you don't know your numbers you can't take care of patients effectively.

Your numbers are your scoreboard.

They are the best way to know whether or not you are winning. Knowing your numbers means you have good metrics that you can look at to see the success of your entire team and you can use them to track your progress towards your goals and your vision.

Here are some key practice statistics and how to use them effectively.

New Patients
I recommend you know your new patients per week and per month. For instance, you should know if you average six new patients per week and you average 26 new patients per month. The average Upper Cervical Doc is seeing about 15 new patients per month based on our surveys.

Patient Visits
It's good to at least know how many people you are helping (otherwise known as patient visits) per week. But it's also helpful to know your patient visits per month. It can also be helpful to know how many patient visits you see per day and even per half day. The average Upper Cervical Doc is seeing about 100 patient visits per week based on our surveys.

Collections
You need to know how much money your practice is collecting. You should definitely know these numbers based on what they are per month, per week, and per day. The average Upper Cervical Doc is collecting about $20,000 per month.

Profit
In addition to knowing how much revenue you are bringing in its also important to know how much you are keeping. A chiropractic practice should strive to have an overhead of 50% or less.

Patient Visit Average (PVA)

The chiropractic industry average PVA is about 15. Most Upper Cervical Doctors have a PVA slightly higher. Let's say about 23. This literally means that the average Upper Cervical Doc is having to look for another new patient to replace the one that just completed 23 visits. If you succeed in replacing the patients that leave, the practice will remain where it is.

On the other hand, a practice with a PVA of 23 will require a great amount of time, energy, and money spent on attracting new ones if you want to experience growth.

Patient Visit Average (PVA) is the average number of visits your patients are coming in to see you. You get this number by adding up all your Patient Visits for at least 8 weeks and then dividing the total Patient Visits by the total New Patients.

For example:

For 8 weeks the number of Patient Visits was 88, 92, 86, 93, 98, 104, 95 & 105. If you add those up you get 761. During the same 8 weeks, your new patients were 3, 4, 3, 5, 6, 3, 4 & 5. The total New Patients would be 33. Patient Visits divided by New Patients is 761 divided by 33 equals 23.1 which can be averaged to 23.

That means your patients are coming to see you an average of 23 times. Some see you once and some see you their entire life, but the average is 23 times.

PVA tells you how well you are doing on patient education and retention.

The better you get at it, the higher your PVA will rise.

Retention is a crucial part of growing the practice of your dreams and is an art that can definitely be mastered. We will talk more about this subject in the retention chapter later in the book.

Office Visit Average (OVA)

OVA is the average amount you are collecting for each visit. You get this number by adding up all your Collections for at least 8 weeks and all your Patient Visits for the same number of weeks and then dividing the total Collections by the total Patient Visits.

To go from $25,000 per month to $38,000 per month you will need to increase your office visit average, your patient visits or both.

For instance, if you were able to increase your office visit average from $60 per visit to $92 per visit while still seeing 95 patient visits per week your average collections would increase from approximately $25,000 per month to $38,000 per month.

Or if your office visit average stayed at $60 per visit and average patient visits per week increased to 150 you would also be collecting about $38,000 per month.

Deciding to increase your prices, see more patients or both will depend on you and your market. Either way, you're going to need more new patients in order to reach the level where you can bring on an associate who can do what you do and give you a level of security and freedom that is impossible to have in a solo practice.

If you want to see 150 Patient Visits you can figure out how many New Patients you need by dividing 150 by your PVA. If it is 23, you need to average 6.5 new patients per week to make your Patient Visits rise to 150.

Average Care Plan

You can also get a more in-depth understanding by keeping track of your care plan recommendations (if you do care plans) for the month and taking an average of those. This is a true average care plan.

Let me give you an example. If you had 15 new patients in a month and your care plan recommendations for those 15 new patients were $2000, $1500, $1800, $1675, $2500, $2250, $2750, $1900, $1200, $2000, $2100, $1800, $1600, $2000, $2200 than your average care plan would be $1951 for the month.

You should be keeping all of these statistics in a spreadsheet for you to review during weekly meetings and planning meetings.

KNOW YOUR NUMBERS:
P&L, BALANCE SHEET, AND DEBT

As a business owner, you need to be able to read a Profit and Loss Statement and Balance Sheet.

A profit and loss can be created by you or your bookkeeper. But either way, you need to know how to read it. Don't just rely on your bookkeeper or CPA…you need to know your numbers. QuickBooks is a very easy way to keep track of a profit and loss and balance sheet. You should be able to get a bookkeeper to do your monthly books, write all your checks and do other bookkeeping tasks for around $100-$300 per month. This is a great investment and should be one of the first things you outsource.

On your profit and loss, you will have a breakdown of your income and your expenses. Your expenses are all of your business overhead. Your income is all of your practice revenue. Your profit is your revenue minus your overhead. As I mentioned earlier your goal is to have 50% or higher profit margin. Meaning that if you collect $30,000 per month than your total overhead should be $15,000 per month or less.

A balance sheet will give you a breakdown of your total assets and debt. All of your equipment and if you own your building should be included on your balance sheet as assets. Any debt that you have including business credit cards, business loans etc. should be listed on your balance sheet as liabilities.

Debt

Taking on debt is one of the ways that many businesses fail. Debt can cause severe consequences for businesses and should be avoided if at all possible. If you are in debt now I highly recommend that you put a plan in place to begin to reduce and eventually completely eliminate your business debt. Your goal should be to have a debt-free practice.

One of the simplest ways to do this is to utilize Dave Ramsey's debt snowball plan and list your debts from smallest to largest and then begin to attack your smallest debt. Once that debt is paid off take whatever you are paying towards that first debt and apply it to your next smallest debt. Once that loan is paid off you move it to your third smallest debt and so on. This debt snowball is an excellent way to build momentum and get out of debt quickly.

Profit First

In the book ***Profit First*** by Mike Michalowicz, he discusses the importance of splitting your revenue into different business bank accounts in order to keep your operations account as small as possible.

The idea behind this is the same as having a small plate when eating in order to eat less. If you keep less money in your operations account you tend to spend less.

One of the simplest ways to do this is just to open 4 different business bank accounts instead of just one at your bank:

1. Operations Account (50%)
2. Tax Account (15%)
3. Owners Compensation Account (20%)
4. Profit Account (15%)

Your operations account will be where you have all of your revenue go and where you have all of your automatic payments set up. Whenever you have your bookkeeping done whether it's once a month or twice a month you're going to transfer money out of your operations account and into your other accounts.

You will keep 50% in your operations account, transfer out 15% of your gross revenue into a tax account, 20% of your gross revenue into an owner's compensation account and 15% of your gross revenue into a profit account. These percentages can be slightly different based on your particular practice situation.

The exception to this would be if you have debt then you want to attack the debt and reduce your profit account and possibly your owner's compensation account percentages depending on how much debt you have.

Here is an example of how it works:

You collected $30,000 this month and all that money is sitting in your bank account that you have called your "Operations Account" (you should be able to add an account nickname in your online banking).

Next, do the following:

- immediately transfer $6000 into your Owners Compensation Account (20% of 30,000)
- immediately transfer $4500 into your Tax Account (15% of 30,000)
- immediately transfer $4500 into your Profit Account (15% of 30,000)

You would then pay yourself out of your owner's compensation account directly by just writing a check to yourself for $6000 at the beginning of the month or whenever you usually pay yourself and depositing that check in your personal checking account.

The profit and tax accounts will just grow as you transfer money into them. You only take money out of your tax account for tax payments whether they are quarterly or end-of-the-year payments. At the end of each quarter take 50% of what you have in your profit account as a bonus and put it into your personal checking account. Just write yourself a nice big bonus check. The other 50% continues to stay in the profit account and grows and is your retained earnings. This is essentially an emergency fund for anything that might happen.

This is a tremendous way to manage the business finances that will allow you to manage your overhead while setting aside money for taxes, owner's compensation, and profit simultaneously.

If you apply the principles in this chapter to have great meetings, great systems and know your numbers it will make a tremendous difference to your practice success.

CHAPTER EIGHT

SET THE STAGE FOR SUCCESS

Upper Cervical Practice Brand Building

*"If you don't give the market the story to talk about,
they'll define your brand's story for you."*

– David Brier

The first step in building your Upper Cervical Practice Brand is defining your ideal patient profile (a.k.a. target market or buyer persona) and your niche, as this will guide you when it comes to building your brand including naming your practice, logo, color scheme, website, marketing etc.

A product or service that is for "everyone" is really for "no one".

Sometimes Upper Cervical Doctors might think if they just focus on a particular ideal patient they will be pushing everyone else away.

The truth is that the best way to dramatically increase your income is to have a well-defined, specific and ideal patient and niche.

The riches are truly in the niches.

Gaining 90% of a niche market is more possible AND more profitable than gaining just 5% of the total market.

WHAT IS A TARGET MARKET?

Business to Community describes target markets like this:

> "A lot of demographic information and very little psychographic information."

This is an example of a target market:

- Gender: Female
- Age: 35-50 years old
- Annual Income: $50,000-90,0000
- Location: Atlanta, Georgia

With that little information are you able to properly find and communicate with prospective new patients?

I don't think so.

An ideal patient profile utilizes the target market demographic information and much more in order to develop a fictionalized representation of the person that you're looking to market to.

Why is this useful?

To be effective in marketing, especially digital marketing, it is important that you know as much as possible about the people that you would like to see more of in your office.

HOW TO DEVELOP AN IDEAL PATIENT PROFILE

Hubspot has some excellent information when it comes to this topic. They discuss a series of 7 questions to ask yourself in order to develop your ideal patient profile. I adapted them into the most important questions for the Upper Cervical Chiropractor to be asking themselves in order to develop their ideal patient profile.

What is their demographic information?

This portion of the target market is still important for you to understand

What does a day in their life look like?

This is a very interesting exercise. Begin by picturing who this ideal patient is and think about their daily life. Is it someone with migraine headaches, who wakes up every morning, not knowing if their day will start with a headache? Is it a young mother who on a daily basis is frustrated and tired because she can't find an answer to her baby's colic? Beginning to picture that person's daily life will really help you with the rest of the questions.

What are their pain points?

You're in business because you're solving a problem for your target audience. How does that problem affect their day to day life? Go into detail and focus on the nuances that illustrate how that problem makes them feel.

What do they value most, and what are their goals?

What is most important to your ideal patient? What are they looking to accomplish? Think about their pain points to better understand their goals.

Where did they go for information?

Where is your ideal patient? Are they online? And if so, where are they online?

What experiences are your ideal patients looking for when investigating or utilizing your service?

Will your ideal patient think you are trustworthy? Will they picture you as credible and knowledgeable about their condition or problem?

What are the most common objections to your service?

Answering common objections for your prospective ideal patients is a key part of building trust and credibility. What are the most common questions that patients have when they 1st come into your office?

After you answer these 7 questions and begin to develop this ideal patient profile, it is important that you share this information with your entire team so that all of you are focused on the types of people that you want to attract into your practice. You want to get as detailed as possible.

Once you have this profile in hand, you can begin to custom craft your unique marketing messages.

Just like with Upper Cervical Chiropractic, the more specific you can be, the better the result will be.

WHAT IS A NICHE?

A niche is a tightly defined portion of a sub-category. For example, our company is Upper Cervical Marketing so we don't work with all

84

chiropractors but only Upper Cervical Chiropractors. This is our ideal client profile "Upper Cervical Chiropractors".

But our niche is the service that we offer to Upper Cervical Chiropractors which is digital marketing services, practice products and business strategies to help them increase new patients, improve referrals, and retention. This is a tightly defined niche.

The target market is the "who"

The niche is the "what you are helping them with"

Once you determine your ideal patient profile you then need to focus on connecting that ideal patient with what you are helping them with by identifying your niche.

Identifying Your Niche

When I was in practice I chose to focus on Upper Cervical Chiropractic specifically the NUCCA technique and I specifically focused on helping women with migraine headaches.

My ideal patient profile was women who were 35 to 55 years old with migraine headaches in my local community and my niche was I corrected the Atlas Subluxation Complex with the NUCCA technique, which was frequently the cause of their migraines.

This focus allowed me to have a very successful cash practice where I was taking care of the people that I wanted to take care of and delivering the service that I knew they needed.

There are many different types of conditions that could make up an ideal patient profile that a doctor can focus on in their practice such as scoliosis, fibromyalgia, migraines, vertigo, pregnancy, colic, ear infections, ADHD, autism, pediatrics etc.

What specific group of people do you want to serve and how are you going to help them?

The key word here is specific. The more specific the better.

Let's take an example, let's say you want to work with people who suffer from vertigo and you want to deliver Blair Upper Cervical Chiropractic.

The general group would be people who suffer from vertigo.

But there are all different types of people who have vertigo symptoms.

For example:

- Ménière's Disease
- dizziness
- disequilibrium
- multiple sclerosis
- whiplash
- post-concussion syndrome
- cochlear hydrops
- tinnitus
- vestibular migraine sufferers

And the list goes on and on and on.

The more you can focus and specify your target market the better you're going to be able to serve them with your niche.

Let's say you decide you really want to focus on people suffering from Ménière's Disease.

Ask yourself these questions:

- Who are these people?
- How old are they?
- What do they care about?
- What kind of injuries do they suffer from?
- What other health professionals interact with them?
- Are there support groups they are part of?
- Are there conferences they attend?

Let's say based on these questions and others you come up with a ideal patient profile that looks like this:

"We serve people suffering from Ménière's Disease who are 35 to 55 years old and care about their quality of life. These people may suffer from head and neck injuries including whiplash, concussion or other injuries affecting the head and neck. Other health professionals that interact with people suffering from Ménière's Disease include neurologists, physical therapists, nutritionists, naturopaths, and general practitioners. There are both online and in person support groups and also conferences that these people may attend. The condition is frequently debilitating and those who suffer from it are looking for answers and results."

Now that you have a great picture of what your ideal patient looks like the next step is to determine how to communicate that your niche of Blair Upper Cervical Chiropractic helps people suffering from this condition improve their quality of life.

This will also help you to focus on who you should be building relationships with including neurologists, physical therapists, general practitioners and others that work with people suffering from Ménière's Disease.

And lastly, this can directly impact your marketing including the images you use on your website, the video testimonials that you accumulate and use in your social media, and the blogs you write. These should all be focused on people with Ménière's Disease and related conditions who want to improve their quality of life through Blair Upper Cervical Chiropractic.

Will you see other types of patients? Absolutely.

But by focusing on a specific ideal patient profile and how to serve them with a specific niche it will allow you to become the go-to doc in your area for your target market AND many others.

Once you determine who your ideal patient is and the niche you are using to serve them the next step is naming (or renaming) your Upper Cervical Practice.

NAMING YOUR UPPER CERVICAL PRACTICE

When choosing the name of your Upper Cervical Practice it is vital that you take into account the possible perceptions and branding implications of your practice name.

Unfortunately, the term Chiropractic or Chiropractor has some negative connotations to a large portion of the public. Chiropractic has a negative brand equity that is hurting the growth of chiropractic in general. Most people are not neutral when it comes to chiropractic – they already have an opinion – and it usually isn't a good one.

According to the 2007 Gallup poll that evaluated ethics and honesty of various professions, chiropractors rank just a couple notches above lawyers and used car salesmen when it comes to the public's perception of the integrity of chiropractors as a whole. Even when the public does have a favorable view of chiropractors – it's exclusively focused on neck and back pain.

This is why it is crucial that you position your practice uniquely in the minds of the public and health practitioners as *Upper Cervical or Craniocervical Junction Specialists* and not *Chiropractic*. Upper Cervical does not have the negative brand equity that Chiropractic does and so many people will give Upper Cervical the benefit of the doubt and not bring their preconceived notions to their decision-making. If you can position Upper Cervical as the unique health care approach that it is separate from Chiropractic in the mind of your community you will have more success when it comes to your marketing, especially if you want to help people with other chronic health conditions besides neck and back pain.

Your practice name is part of your subconscious communication online just as much as your practice logo, color scheme, and social proof factors. All of your branding should represent your unique Upper Cervical Approach and be congruent with who you and your practice are. According to some studies you only have about 50 milliseconds to make a first impression online.

Be aware that in some areas Chiropractors must have the word Chiropractic in their name. So, check with your board before naming your practice. If it is at all possible you want to stay away from the word Chiropractic when choosing a name for your practice.

3 Common Naming Mistakes

One of the mistakes that we see is doctors naming their practices such obscure names that prospective patients will never know what it means. So resist the urge to name your company after the mythical Greek god of health or the Latin phrase for "We're number one!"

If a name has a natural, intuitive sound and a special meaning, it can work. If it's too complex and puzzling, it will remain a mystery to your potential patients.

Another mistake is doctors originally choosing the wrong name and then refusing to change it. Many clinic owners know they have a problem with their name and just hope it will somehow magically resolve itself. Although it is a pain to change your name to match your branding and marketing it can certainly pay off in the end. Just make sure that you change all of your directory listings so Google knows that your name has changed.

The last mistake that we commonly see is getting the "committee" involved in your decision. We live in a democratic society, and it seems like the right thing to do–to involve everyone (your friends, family, employees, and patients) in an important decision.

A better method is to involve only the key decision-makers–the fewer the better–and select only the people you feel have the company's best interests at heart. The need for personal recognition can skew results, so you'll be best served by those who can park their egos at the door. Also, make sure you have some right-brain types in the mix. Get too many left brains on board, and your name will most likely end up too literal and descriptive.

Choosing Your Practice Name

When choosing a practice name, keep the following tips in mind:

- Choose a name that appeals not only to you but also to the kind of patients you are trying to attract (your ideal patient).
- Choose a comforting or familiar name that conjures up pleasant memories so potential patients respond to your business on an emotional level.
- Don't pick a name that is long or confusing.
- Be careful with having your last name in your practice name (i.e. Smith Spinal Care). If you ever want to sell your practice to someone else or have associates having your last name in your practice can be detrimental.

Good words to include in your name to reach your target market may include:

Precision	Specific
Balance	Posture
Life	Health
Spinal	Center

Complete	Care
Precise	Balanced
Advanced	Vital
Upper Cervical	Spine
Health Clinic	Spine Center
Technique Name (i.e. NUCCA, Atlas Orthogonal, Blair etc.)	City Name (i.e. Dallas) or Area (i.e. Apple Valley)

Here are some good examples of Upper Cervical Practice names:

- Precision Spine Clinic
- Houston Specific
- Complete Balance
- Upper Cervical Toledo
- Advanced Spinal Care
- NUCCA Health Clinic
- Vital Posture Clinic

Once you determine the name of your practice or the new name of your practice you can then begin building a branding strategy around the name including your logo, color scheme, website, online marketing, business cards, brochures and office decor.

THE IMPACT OF YOUR LOGO AND COLOR SCHEME

When marketing your Upper Cervical Practice, it is essential that you choose the right colors and design elements in your logo, website, marketing collateral and color scheme that is congruent with your ideal patient profile that we discussed in the last section.

The primary individual that you are focused on attracting into your practice will have a major impact on the color scheme, logo, and website design.

If your target market is families, for instance, you want to focus your colors on those that will attract 30 to 50-year-old women as they are the primary decision-makers when it comes to health care decisions for their families.

If you are looking to attract hockey players into your practice then you would use a color scheme that was focused on that target demographic.

Another aspect to keep in mind is a particular market. Certain markets may be more connected to certain color schemes. Understanding your market and the culture that surrounds your practice is crucial.

Here are some general recommendations that will work in most markets based on the most common demographic in Upper Cervical Chiropractic Practices which is 35 to 55-year-old Caucasian women. You will want to adapt this to match your ideal patient profile.

Logos

When you are having someone create a logo for your Upper Cervical Practice it is very important that you give specific instructions related to your ideal patient profile, color scheme, and your Upper Cervical Approach.

Having images that focus on the head and neck relationship that is so vital to health and to your practice makes sense. Instead of just another Chiropractic logo with a version of a spine in it, differentiate yourself beginning at your logo.

Website Color Scheme

In a study that evaluated the Impact of Color in Marketing, researchers found that up to 90% of snap judgments made about products and services can be based on color alone.

You don't have to be a website designer but a good question to ask yourself is whether your website colors are drawing people in or pushing them away?

When it comes to the color scheme of your website here are some basic recommendations about website colors:

- Limit the number of colors to no more than 3, this will reduce visual clutter.
- Use colors that will suit your website, its function and the message to your ideal patient.
- Avoid harsh colors by adding texture and natural tones.
- Colors should not clash, instead, they should complement each other and make the important information stand out.
- Colored text needs to be legible on a contrasting color background.
- Avoid backgrounds that are too bold, busy and colorful.

- Be careful when using light text on a darker background.
- Avoid neon and fluorescent lighting.

When it comes to Upper Cervical Chiropractic color schemes in logos and websites and other marketing collateral there are 4 colors that tend to be the most effective when focusing on the most common demographic:

- Blues
- Yellows
- Greens
- Purples

Blue is a very calming, cool and serene color. Subtle blues are often used to indicate professionalism, credibility, and trustworthiness. Light tones are a great option for a calm background. Blue also offers and creates feelings of trust. However, too bright and bold blues can appear as too much. Too much blue can also cause things to feel cold.

Yellow is an uplifting color that leaves you feeling lighter and happier. Seeing yellow elevates moods and refreshes the brain cells. This energetic color is thought to emit warmth and nourishment. Yellow is said to stimulate mental activity, muscular energy and attracts attention. However, too much yellow can put a strain on the eyes and bring about anxiety.

Green is an earthy tone that will leave your viewers feeling regenerated and it has physical healing properties. Green is also believed to lower blood pressure, calm the mind and stimulate creativity. Using too dark a shade of green can leave your website looking and feeling cramped.

Purple is a very influential and spiritual color. It oozes royalty, dignity, energy, extravagance and high aspirations.

In order to ensure you are getting the best possible results with your online and offline marketing for your Upper Cervical Practice, it is important to pick a color scheme and logo that properly represents your brand and attracts your ideal patient.

Bringing It All Together

Once you have identified your ideal patient profile, determined your niche, and created your practice name, logo, and color scheme, then you want to put it all together on your website and other online properties.

We will get more detailed on websites in chapter 15 but for now, just make sure that you are thinking through how to integrate all of these different aspects together on your website. Once the website is created, it is important to have a consistent color scheme, logo, pictures etc. on your Facebook page, Instagram, YouTube, Pinterest and other social networks.

POSTERS, CHARTS, BROCHURES, AND MORE

Your in-office presence is just as important as your online presence when it comes to your branding. Once again designing your office around your ideal patient is key. Utilizing a consistent color scheme, logo, pictures etc. that are consistent with your online presence is also important. If you are an Upper Cervical Doctor then it is absolutely crucial that you are properly branding yourself throughout your online and offline presence. It certainly isn't congruent to have brochures or other educational products in your office showing general Chiropractic procedures.

It's especially not good for one of your patients to take a general Chiropractic brochure from your office to a friend, and then try to explain that you do something different than what's in the brochure!

The types of brochures that you use, the types of pictures you have on your walls, the types of educational materials you use, and even the types of charts you have should all be consistent with your ideal patient profile, niche, and branding.

Brochures

A great source for Upper Cervical Specific brochures is www.uppercervicalstuff.com.

I really like these brochures. They offer 16 different condition brochures that contain the latest Upper Cervical Research and our very congruent with upper cervical (no pictures of rotary breaks).

Brochures include:

- Asthma
- Carpal Tunnel
- Depression
- Diabetes

- Digestive Disorders
- Ear Infections
- Fibromyalgia
- High Blood Pressure
- Inner Ear Disorders
- Low Back Pain
- Migraine Headaches
- Multiple Sclerosis
- Seizure Disorders & Epilepsy
- Sleep Disorders
- TMJ
- Trigeminal Neuralgia (TN)

Posters and Charts

Visual learners are the largest group within your practice and visual demonstrations using pictures, images, and spatial understanding are critical to effective patient learning.

You can find some excellent posters that demonstrate the Upper Cervical Misalignment for you to utilize in your report of findings that make a tremendous impact on visual learners in our online store at www.uppercervicalmarketing.com/shop including many posters that are consistent with an Upper Cervical Practice Branding Strategy including:

- The Effects of the Upper Cervical Misalignment Poster
- Posture Changes from an Upper Cervical Misalignment Poster
- The Upper Cervical Misalignment and the Brain Poster

Utilizing these images as you describe the impact of the Upper Cervical Misalignment on the health and life of your new or existing patients can be extremely effective.

Great branding is all about connecting with your ideal patient in an integrated and cohesive way. Once you identify your ideal patient profile and the niche you are going to use to serve them you can then design an effective branding strategy for both online and off-line use.

CHAPTER NINE

BECOME A MASTER COMMUNICATOR

Seamlessly Communicate during Your Consult, Exam, Report of Findings and Other Patient Communication

"What we've got here is failure to communicate."

– Paul Newman in Cool Hand Luke

Mastering communication is a critical characteristic of top Upper Cervical Doctors.

Great communication skills can be learned and applied in your practice.

Communication begins with the first phone conversation with your team and carries through every interaction between you and your patients.

In this chapter, we are going to investigate the different areas of communication within your practice including:

- phone communication
- welcoming the new patient
- consultation
- examination
- taking x-rays
- report of findings
- group communication
- visit by visit interactions
- progress exam communication
- re-reports
- care plans
- common mistakes

PHONE COMMUNICATION

Doctors should avoid answering their own phones if at all possible. Patients do not expect doctors to answer the phone, which is why the top Upper Cervical Doctors will train their front desk receptionist, office manager, and other team members to answer the phone effectively. This is one of the areas that are important to constantly role-play and train with your team on a weekly basis.

You have to train your team to be adept at controlling the conversation immediately.

The first thing to keep in mind is the question principle.

He who asks the questions is in control of the conversation.

When your front desk receptionist answers the phone and immediately starts answering questions instead of asking them, then the patient is in complete control of the conversation. If that happens, the patient is much more likely to talk themselves out of coming into your office.

Unfortunately, someone that is sick and suffering and needs your care also has a number of internal barriers that will keep them from coming into your practice and getting the help they need. Your job is to train your team to break down these barriers and allow the patient to get out of their own way so you can help them.

Context is everything when it comes to patient communication.

It would be foolish to tell a patient over the phone that your average care plan is $2000 before they have ever been to your office, met you personally, or before they understand the extent of their problem and how you plan to address it.

Mastering communication means mastering context.

Certain conversations should be done at certain times and not before.

It is important for you to train your team with the initial goal in mind of scheduling the potential new patient for an initial consultation or initial evaluation.

The phone is not the place to discuss all of your fees and all possible scenarios with a potential new patient. Instead, the phone is about connecting with the new patient on a personal level and bringing them into your office to see if you can help them.

Let's look at a few scenarios:

A Potential New Patient Phone Call

There are several questions the new patient caller needs to get answered in their own mind before making an initial appointment including:

1. Does this office give me confidence?
2. Is this doctor experienced?
3. Does this doctor have experience helping people with my problem?
4. Does this office care about me?
5. Is my problem serious?
6. How much will I have to pay?

The first five questions must be addressed before we answer number six.

However, the sixth question is almost always the first question asked by potential new patients!

Your team's phone answering technique should be short and to the point, giving the caller the impression that you are busy, yet professional.

Their voices should be pleasant and upbeat.

Below is just an example. The important thing is to train your front desk receptionist to think on her feet and not just be a robot who repeats a script, rather have certain milestones that she should always hit with a new patient.

The first thing we need to know is how the patient happened to call our office in particular.

Was it from a referral, from the Internet, professional referral, or some other type of marketing?

CA: "Precision Spinal Care, this is Susan I can help you."

PATIENT: "Hello, I was wondering how much you charge for a visit."

CA: "I'd be happy to discuss that with you, but can I get a little information first?"

PATIENT: "Yes, go ahead."

CA: "Can I get your name and phone number just in case we get disconnected?"

PATIENT: "Yes, this is Linda Smith and my phone number is 723-555-8724."

CA: "Excellent, thank you for that. How did you hear about our office? Were you referred by a patient of ours or another doctor?"
(This question gives the caller the idea that most of your new patients come from referrals or professional referrals, and it helps to instill confidence.)

PATIENT: "I was just looking through Facebook and saw some information about your office."

CA: "Oh great that's exciting that you found us on Facebook. Can you tell me what kind of problem you're having, and how long you've had it, Ms. Smith?"

PATIENT: "I've had migraine headaches for about two years and they have been getting more frequent. They are now happening several times per week and when I get them I'm in so much pain and I don't think I can stand it much longer. I'm finding it difficult to work, I can't concentrate, and I need help! I've been to my doctor but he just gave me painkillers and they don't even seem to be working anymore. I feel like I'm in a fog and it's not helping anyway."

CA: "What we have to do is get to the cause of your problem, not just cover it up with drugs. After a while, they cause problems with your stomach and elsewhere. We have a lot of experience helping people get to the cause of migraines. Are you getting any dizziness yet?"

PATIENT: "Yes, it is beginning to do that when I get them. Is that bad?"

CA: "I can tell you that symptoms like yours shouldn't be ignored. It definitely sounds like a problem that we help people with all the time. Our office offers a free migraine consultation. You can come in and meet with our doctor and determine if he can help you. Then, you can decide if you feel comfortable with Dr. Davis and our office."

PATIENT: "I think I'd like to do that. How soon can you see me?"

CA: "Even though we are a busy office, patients who are suffering like you are a priority and we always keep space in our schedule for patients in pain. I have an appointment available at two this afternoon. Can you come then?"

PATIENT: "Yes."
(Give directions to your clinic, send the patient to your website to get your new patient paperwork, and advise the patient about the approximate length of visit.)

CA: "You have an appointment today at 2:00 PM. I really hope we can help you. It's terrible that you're suffering. Again, my name is Susan. I look forward to meeting you."

PATIENT: "Thank you, Susan, you've been very helpful. I'll see you at two o'clock. Goodbye"

CA: You're welcome. Goodbye."

WELCOMING A NEW PATIENT

You only get one opportunity to make a first impression and it is possible for your office to ruin your connection with the new patient before you even meet them.

After your team has spoken with a potential new patient on the phone the next step is to make sure that you give the new patient a WOW experience from the moment they arrive in your office. Making sure that your office is warm, friendly and inviting involves many different factors including:

- the music
- the smells
- the office temperature
- the colors of the walls
- the flooring
- the lighting
- the pictures

It is important to consider all of these subconscious factors when it comes to your lobby environment.

Next, the goal for your front desk receptionist should be to make eye contact and smile as quickly as possible when the new patient enters the office.

I recommend teaching your receptionist to get up and shake hands with the new patient out in the lobby and ask them if they would like some water or tea.

Hopefully, your new patient paperwork is on your website and the patient has completed it before they have come to your office which will make their first visit much more efficient. But if not, you can have your front desk receptionist help them complete the paperwork or give it to them to complete.

Next, the new patient should be taken on a quick tour of the office and then placed in the consultation room.

CONSULTATION, EXAMINATION, TAKING X-RAYS, AND REPORT OF FINDINGS (YOUR SALES PROCESS)

Connecting with the new patient during the consultation, examination, taking x-rays, and report of findings will frequently make all the difference in whether this new patient will become a long-term member of your practice or not.

In other types of businesses, this type of process would be referred to as your sales process and it is just the same in an Upper Cervical Practice…this is your sales process.

Every practice has a sales process whether you like it or not.

When money is being exchanged for a product or service a sales process has taken place.

Sales are vital to the existence of your practice.

If someone is not buying what you have to offer then you are not going to be in practice for very long.

There are many factors that go into connecting well during your sales process including:

- your handshake
- your body language
- your voice inflection
- how you are dressed
- how you smell
- your hair
- your weight
- the patient's learning style
- the patient's personality
- how effectively you use technology
- your passion for your work

The consultation, exam, and report of findings are critical to success in practice.

As Dr. Todd Osborne said in episode 17 of the Upper Cervical Marketing Podcast **"it's the foundation of everything that you're going to do in your practice from day one right on through a lifetime of care for that patient."**

It Starts with Passion

Good communication with patients during your consultation, exam, and report of findings will always start with passion. The more confident, certain and passionate you are about your work the better you can communicate with new and existing patients.

Dr. Dennis Young and Dr. Todd Osborne and I have discussed this on separate podcasts.

You have to believe in what you do and why you do it to have passion.

Your practice is important. The work you do is valuable.

And you have the opportunity to make a difference in the life of every person that walks in your door.

In chapter 2, we discussed the importance of enthusiasm in building a mindset that wins.

Ty Howard said:

> *"Enthusiasm for the job puts passion in the work"*

This is very true. Enthusiasm and passion are intimately connected.

Stephen Covey put it this way:

> *"Passion is the fire, enthusiasm, and courage that an individual feels when she is doing something she loves while accomplishing worthy ends"*

When you cultivate enthusiasm, you will cultivate passion and that will translate into your communication.

Jesus said it this way:

> *"for out of the abundance of the heart his mouth speaks"*

If you truly believe in what you do and are passionate and enthusiastic in your heart, then that is what will come out of your mouth.

DON'T TALK TO EVERY PATIENT THE SAME

Every patient is unique.

This is why scripts can be difficult.

Every script will not work for every person because every person has a unique personality and learning style. The better you can understand personality types and learning styles the better you will be able to communicate with each individual person whether you are using a script or not.

Understanding Personality Styles

In chapter 6 we discussed the importance of understanding personalities as it applies to team dynamics but personality types are also very important when communicating with patients during your consultation and report of findings.

Dr. Jeff Scholten and I discussed this in episode one of the Upper Cervical Marketing Podcast here are some paraphrased quotes from that conversation:

Dr. Scholten says "As an example, when I do my report of findings, I start out by asking:

"If a zero is I've already talked too much and a ten is teach me everything you know, how much do you want to know about what's going on with yourself?"

Their answer will either be:

"I don't need to know much, tell me the basics."

"Tell me everything."

"Based on their answer I will try to zone in on that.

And I will tell them:

"If I tell you too much, try to glaze your eyes over and I'll try to pick up on the non-verbal."

Dr. Scholten continues "It's about matching the patient's personality. So when systems are too non-flexible and unadaptable then there are problems as well. As you're making systems, be cautious about overdoing it in terms of the rigor of it but being very rigorous in terms of having something for everything."

"It's so key to understand patients' personality types. Even a set of paperwork that's filled out by hand can help you identify what their personality style is. Are they writing really, really quickly? Are they missing information? Or is their handwriting completely meticulous? When you have somebody who has all this information on this one piece of paper with meticulous handwriting, this suggests they are analytical. They will likely want the small details. If somebody has crossed three things out and left things blank, you probably don't need to tell them much of anything. Just get them in and get them out. The more you talk the less likely they are to start care because

you're annoying them. So, let's not annoy people. Let's not be weird." Dr. Scholten said.

"The key is your ability to match other people's social styles and move in between social styles effortlessly. The more you can do that and match the type of person you're interacting with at the moment the more successful you will be at giving that person a great experience. And that's something that I think we forget as we're working so hard to make the patient understand what we want to share with them. **We have it backward. We need to share with them what they want to understand.** And it's really about, do they have a problem? Do you think you can help them? Do they want you to try to help them? And if they do, you go forward and you try to help them." Dr. Scholten said.

Understanding Learning Styles

Along with personality styles, it is also important to understand learning styles. The word Doctor means "to teach" and the more effectively you can help patients learn the better you will be at communication.

In episode 52 of the podcast, I discussed the importance of understanding your patients learning styles with Dr. Andy Gibson.

Dr. Gibson has a Master's in Education and has been able to apply much of what he learned in his communication with patients.

Let's take a look at the different learning styles and how to utilize them when communicating with patients.

There are 7 ways that human beings learn information. These 7 learning styles are:

1. **Visual** (spatial): prefer using pictures, images, and spatial understanding.
2. **Auditory** (musical): prefer using sound and music.
3. **Verbal** (linguistic): prefer using words, both in speech and writing.
4. **Physical** (kinesthetic): prefer using your body, hands, and sense of touch.
5. **Logical** (mathematical): prefer using logic, reasoning, and systems
6. **Social** (interpersonal): prefer to learn in groups or with other people.
7. **Solitary** (intrapersonal): prefer to work alone and use self-study.

According to recent research visual learners are the largest group. This is important for you to understand when working with new patients to communicate ideas and understanding related to Upper Cervical Care. When conducting your report of findings with new patients the more effectively you can utilize visual demonstrations of the Upper Cervical Misalignment the better.

One of the best ways to connect with those visual learners while at the same time utilizing the latest technology is with Dr. Kerry Johnson's My Misalignment Software https://mymisalignment.com/. Dr. Johnson has developed a software that can actually create an animation of the patient's misalignment and how your specific Upper Cervical Technique will go about correcting it. It's a very innovative software and it's a great way to communicate Upper Cervical during your report of findings. The software can also be a very effective tool for a patient to communicate what's going on with them to their spouse if they are not at the report. But you also want to keep in mind the other learning styles. We tend to default to our own learning style when presenting information so it's important for you to understand what your learning style is so you know your tendencies. If you don't already know your learning style you can take a learning style quiz for free https://www.learning-styles-online.com/inventory/questions.php.

Let's take a look at how you can utilize each of the 7 learning styles in your practice to effectively communicate Upper Cervical.

Visual Learners
As the largest group within your practice, visual demonstrations using software, pictures, images, charts, videos, and spatial understanding are critical to effective patient learning.

We have some excellent posters in our store that demonstrate the Upper Cervical Misalignment for you to utilize in your report of findings and other patient communication that make a tremendous impact on visual learners. You get any of these at http://uppercervicalmarketing.com/shop/.

Here are some of my favorites:

- The Effects of the Upper Cervical Misalignment Poster
- Posture Changes from an Upper Cervical Misalignment Poster
- The Upper Cervical Misalignment and the Brain Poster
- Blood Flow through the Upper Cervical Spine Poster

Utilizing these images as you describe the impact of the Upper Cervical Misalignment on the health and life of your new patient can be extremely effective.

When conducting progress exams and also during your report of findings I would recommend a chart from Dr. Noel Lloyd that we also have available in our store.

The three phases chart is excellent at communicating how Upper Cervical Care helps a person find fast relief, maximum recovery, and long-lasting results.

Using these types of posters and charts is a great way to connect with visual learners during your report of findings and progress exams.

Auditory Learners
Connecting with auditory learners can be a little more challenging. Auditory learners prefer using sound and music to learn, they essentially learn by listening.

While I would never suggest that you sing your report of findings there are some ways that you can nurture this learning style.

The tone of voice that you use, your voice pace, and your voice inflection can have a dramatic impact on auditory learners actually remembering what you say.

Stay away from monotone.

Changing your tone of voice, sometimes talking faster in order to encourage excitement and lowering your voice to emphasize certain points of your report of findings can all be effective with auditory learners.

You can also help stimulate your auditory learners by having music playing in the office to set a particular tone.

Auditory learners will often need you to talk them through the cause or program extensively.

Verbal Learners
A verbal learner needs to say it themselves in order to understand it. It's important to ask questions in your report of findings for all learning styles but especially verbal learners.

They need to be able to talk it out in order to truly understand it.

Some of the best questions to ask throughout your report of findings are:

- "does that make sense"
- "can you understand how…"
- "describe to me what you understand so far"
- "what questions do you have so far"

As you work with a primary verbal learner in your report of findings, follow-up visits, and progress exams it is important that you consistently ask questions and allow them to essentially teach themselves what you are attempting to communicate.

Kinesthetic Learners
Kinesthetic learners are physical learners meaning that they need to physically feel what you're saying in order to truly understand it.

Ways to connect with kinesthetic learners include demonstrating something within your own body such as a head tilt or other postural changes and then having them create the same postural change and feel how that impacts their body as well.

Kinesthetic learners also do well with handheld models where you can show them anatomy and then have them feel the models themselves.

Logical Learners
Logical learners prefer using logic, reasoning, and systems to understand a new topic.

If you are a logical learner it will be very easy for you to communicate with others who are also driven by understanding through logic, reasoning, and systems but if you are not it's important for you to know that so you can change the way you communicate in these circumstances.

This is again why it's important to understand what kind of learner you are.

Upper Cervical Chiropractic is extremely logical and it will make a tremendous amount of sense to logical learners. Using visual demonstrations like the posters and charts we talked about above while also showing the patient their own x-rays is extremely effective at communicating with logical learners.

Social Learners

Social learners prefer to learn in groups or with other people. These individuals are ideal participants in your healthcare classes (patient orientation class). A good patient orientation class will also encapsulate all of the other learning styles that we discussed so far.

If you are not currently doing a new patient orientation class I would highly recommend that you do one on a consistent basis (ideally one time per week or at least one time per month).

Here are some resources from our online store at www.uppercervicalmarketing.com/shop to help you:

- Creating a New Patient Orientation Class Step-By-Step Kit
- New Patient Orientation Class Audio Demonstration

Solitary Learners

Solitary learners prefer to work alone and use self-study. These are patients that would appreciate a booklet so they can continue to learn and educate others on their own.

Once again in our store, we have a tremendous resource to help with your solitary learners which is an eight-page Upper Cervical Specific Report of Findings Booklet http://uppercervicalmarketing.com/product/upper-cervical-specific-report-findings-booklets/.

Knowing how patients learn and also knowing that many people will have a mix of many of these styles is an important part of effectively communicating Upper Cervical to both new and existing patients.

INDIVIDUALIZED REPORT OF FINDINGS AND CARE PLANS

In episode 3 of the Upper Cervical Marketing Podcast, I discussed in detail how Dr. Robert Brooks performs his report of findings and creates individualized care plans based on the misalignment pattern of the patient.

Dr. Brooks has a tremendous seminar that goes much deeper into the concepts in this section called *Taking Care of People*. If you have not been to his class before I highly recommend it.

You can find more information at http://www.tcopseminar.com/.

In our conversation, Dr. Brooks explained that there are five questions you must answer for a new patient during your report of findings:

1. **Can you help me?**
2. **What is IT? (How you describe the subluxated spine)**
3. **Do I have IT?**
4. **How is IT affecting me?**
5. **What do I need to do to take care of IT?**

Here are some paraphrased quotes about how he answers these questions from the interview.

"**Dr. Brooks:** …on the follow-up visit, we'll have the person come in and actually sit down with the doctor and we go through and show them 'This is what a spine misalignment looks like. This is what happens if it's misaligned over time.

Then we go through their own X-rays showing them their misalignment, matching with the body distortions, the short legs, the twisting in the body frame that we've measured on an Anatometer. Then, we make the first correction and take a set of post-X-ray's and review those.

Now, once we've done that and we read the post-X-rays and release the patient, we don't talk about a care plan until the next visit. **Our care plans are designed based on the patient's situation and everyone's care plan is different.**"

Dr. Brooks continues: "Our initial care plan is for 90 days, and we explain to our patients that there are **5 different categories of misalignments** including:

1. **small and simple**
2. **big and simple**
3. **small with a complication**
4. **big with a complication**
5. **very complicated**

(*Orthogonally based UC Doctors see note below)

*When we look at the set of pre-X-rays in an Orthogonal-based Upper Cervical practice, what we have is the ability to determine if this is a simple misalignment. With NUCCA, which is what my foundation is now; misalignments are type 1, 2, 3 or 4. So, 1, 2, 3 would be simple. A 4 would be a complication. There is one misalignment with another one on top of it for example. So now, those are either going to be small, or they're going to be large; and, of course, I would expect a small simple misalignment to be more stable than a large complicated misalignment for example." Dr. Brooks said.

"We also explain that their <u>pattern of stability</u> will be one of the following 5 categories:

- **Category 1** misalignments correct to normal initially and stay in alignment really well (most stable)
- **Category 2** misalignments correct to normal initially but come out of alignment several times before the body is strong enough to stabilize them
- **Category 3** misalignments will only <u>reduce</u> initially, and then come out of alignment and then reduce some more and come out and reduce some more until it eventually corrects and stabilizes
- **Category 4** misalignments are able to <u>reduce</u> but not correct completely
- **Category 5** misalignments are not able to be reduced at all.

I've worked with 25,000 spines over 40 years and there have been only 47 people for which I have not been able to reduce the misalignment at all."

Dr. Brooks continues **"And so, by knowing what I'm working with and being able to have integrity with the patient when I tell them what their misalignment is and what I'm able to do with it, it actually creates more of a compliance or more of an involvement in their care.** So, those things are simply fundamental to creating care plans based on an individual basis. So that everybody doesn't get the same plan. **They're getting a care plan based on their misalignment and their pattern of stability."**

Dr. Brooks continues "After the initial 90 days, the patient goes through 6-8 months of stability care to maximize recovery of the ligaments and tendons. Then, they are monitored for one month for every year the spine was misaligned, and then eventually into wellness care.

This creates a model for patient care to transition into a lifetime patient."

COMMON MISTAKES DURING YOUR CONSULTATION, EXAM, AND REPORT

Dr. Todd Osborne and I discussed in detail in episode 17 common mistakes doctors make during their consultation, exam and report and I want to outline some of those here.

Consultation Mistakes

Letting a consult go too long. You can do a fantastic consultation in 7 to 10 minutes. If your consult is going 30 to 45 minutes you have lost all authority and control of the situation.

Making it an interrogation, not a conversation. There is an art to asking questions in a friendly way that promotes likability rather than the patient feeling that you are peppering them with questions during an interrogation.

Turning a consult into a report of findings. Context is king when it comes to your consultation, exam, and report. Don't get ahead of yourself and start explaining everything to them during the consultation. During the consultation, you should be focused on being an ear, not a mouth.

Promising results. You should never tell a patient during a consultation that you can help them. You could tell them that you're going to do everything possible to find out if you can help them but you don't want to promise results or get ahead of yourself before you do the exam, take your films and do your full analysis.

Exam Mistakes

Doing way too many tests. The key focus of the exam is to determine whether or not the person has signs of an atlas subluxation complex. You need to have basic tests that will determine whether or not a subluxation is present and then move on to the next step which is taking the proper x-rays. This is not the time to do every orthopedic and neurological test that you learned in chiropractic school.

Taking way too much time. Again, a common mistake is having your exam go on and on for 30 minutes or longer. Be efficient, get the information that you need and move on to the films.

Remember the context. The exam is not your report of findings. You can certainly do some basic education about what the tests determine but don't get lost in the details and spend 15 minutes explaining all of the results of the tests.

Report Mistakes

Too complicated. One of the most common mistakes doctors make during the report is they get overly technical and lose the patient. Keep it simple. The best reports are usually done in a way that a second-grader could understand what's happening.

Too long. Another very common mistake during the report of findings is just talking way too much. During the consultation, you are the ear. During the exam, you are the eye. And during the report, you are the mouth but this is not the time to give them your entire healthcare class. Ask questions, engage with the patient and help them understand on a basic level so that they can make a wise decision. The most important things to communicate are what's the problem and can you help.

Minimizing the problem. Another common mistake is not communicating the seriousness of the subluxation. It's not about scaring them but it is about communicating that the problem that they have is doing significant damage to their brain and body and needs to be corrected.

Learn from these great doctors, avoid these mistakes and lay the foundation for a great practice during your consultation, exam and report.

COMMUNICATING TO GROUPS

Dr. Corinne Weaver is a master at group communication and building community. In episode five of the podcast, we discussed a variety of topics focused around group communication and educational classes here are some paraphrased sections from the podcast.

Dr. Weaver: "Our office has new patients attend a dinner and class before they meet the doctor one-on-one. My staff says "Before you meet Dr. Weaver, we have a class for you to attend with your spouse called Ask the Doctor."
When they come I tell them about upper cervical and my story. I tell them patient testimonials. I have a PowerPoint presentation that I go through.

We feed them dinner. I give them myself for 45 minutes, and then they make an appointment.

My consultation is $125. If they come to the dinner, we knock it down to $69. So, it's beneficial for them to come to the dinner and get the discounted consult."

Dr. Weaver continues: "Topics I cover include:

- Why do I do the scans?
- Why do I do upper cervical?
- Why do you check my leg length?
- What are you looking for in the x-ray?

We have a variety of other educational classes including:

- nutrition classes
- how to make healthy choices when grocery shopping class
- stress management classes
- detox classes"

Another terrific resource when it comes to group communication is Keith Wassung. Keith has been a chiropractic advocate and lay lecturer for over 30 years and has done thousands of lectures about chiropractic to the public.

In episode 34 of the podcast, we discussed common mistakes that doctor's make when doing group lectures and how to do them effectively.

Here are some excerpts from that conversation.

"Dr. Davis: So Keith, doctors are doing lectures all the time in their office, outside of their office, what are some of the most common mistakes that you see doctors making when they're doing lectures?

Keith Wassung: "Well, I think the big mistake is, **they go in with the mindset that I'm here to get new patients**. Now, getting new patients is the natural result of it, but if that's the primary objective, you are actually going to turn the majority of people off.

So, to counteract that, we're going to go in with 4 objectives.

1. To change their thought process about health, how their body works with Upper Cervical Chiropractic being an option.

113

2. To get them so concerned, excited, and aware about their nervous system's potential for possibly solving their problem and improving their life that the next logical step in their mind is to get checked.
3. To get them to take home information that they can read.
4. Leveraging that lecture into more lectures."

Keith continues: "I want them to take home data. The information they can read from mainstream physiology journals and say, 'Wow! This is even more impressive than the guy said.' They need to hear it again and have the ability to pass the information on to others.

When you are finishing up hand out a feedback sheet, and say, 'Folks you're probably wondering if we do other lectures? Yes, we actually do several other talks. We lecture on kids, sports, etc. If you're part of a group, whether it's your church group or where you work, a family reunion, or just six friends for lunch and you would find this information valuable then put it down on the sheet and we'll see if we can accommodate it."

Keith has some terrific Upper Cervical Educational Materials for doing presentations and handouts that you can get at www.keithwassung.com.

To take a deeper dive into the principles laid out in this chapter and the entire book go to http://uppercervicalpracticemastery.com/academy to learn more about the companion course that goes along with this *Upper Cervical Practice Mastery* book. The companion course contains in-depth webinars about each chapter, email Q&A, and exclusive access to a private Facebook group for accountability and community with other doctors and students looking to become Upper Cervical Practice Masters.

CHAPTER TEN

KEEP PATIENTS ON TRACK

The Importance of Progress Exams

"It does not matter how slow you go as long as you do not stop."

– Confucius

Progress exams are an absolute necessity for a top Upper Cervical Doctor. Doing consistent and effective progress exams can help you in many ways including:

- improve retention
- increase referrals
- increase video testimonials
- increase online reviews
- keep you excited and motivated
- inspire and encourage your team
- identify issues before they get worse

Doing consistent progress exams with every patient is one of the most effective ways to do **retention marketing**. Most everyone knows about internal and external marketing but there is a third type of marketing for the Upper Cervical Practice and that is retention marketing to retain the patients you already have. It is much easier to keep a patient then is to get a new patient. Therefore, your team should be focusing on retention-based marketing on a daily, weekly and monthly basis.

HOW TO DO A GOOD PROGRESS EXAM

By consistently doing a progress exam with your patients every 10 to 12 visits you will keep them engaged in their healing process and their overall progress. Patients forget how unhealthy they were when they started care. Progress exams help them to take a realistic look at how far they have come and is a great opportunity for you to remind them of the potential benefits they will receive from continuing care.

I also recommend the progress exam include a form for them to complete that asks them questions which help them reflect on all the ways that their body has changed since they have been under care. I also recommend that the doctor perform objective evaluations to measure progress.

The combination of the subjective and the objective during the progress exam can be a very powerful combination in promoting patient retention and referrals.

A good progress exam should be:

- **Consistent** (every 10 to 12 visits)
- **Subjective Component** (use a feedback form that discusses their original complaints but also other health benefits derived from care including sleep, energy, digestion improvements, etc.)
- **Objective Component** (perform many or all objective tests that were done at the beginning of care in order to compare and measure progress)

WAYS TO USE THE INFORMATION GATHERED DURING PROGRESS EXAMS

Obtain Social Proof

When it becomes evident during the progress exam that your patient is beginning to get results, it is important for you to help them put their results into words so they can tell others about their story.

One of the best ways you can do that is by having them complete an online review on Google, Facebook or Yelp. This will help them to organize their thoughts about what has taken place in their body since they began care while at the same time improving your ability to attract more patients from the Internet.

Another way that you can teach them to testify is by having them do a video testimonial. Once again this will highlight in their mind how far they have come. Their video testimonial will also allow you to reach more people who need your help when you distribute and promote it online.

If you can develop effective ways to obtain online reviews and video testimonials during progress exams, it will pay off for years to come. Here are a few ideas some doctors have used to motivate their patients to give reviews and/or video testimonials:

- Offer a gift card
- Offer a free product/service your office provides
- Have a "Thank you" box with items patients can choose from (gift card, gifts with your office name and contact information on them: water bottle, coffee mugs, pens, keychain lights, etc.)

Identify Issues

Another important benefit of doing progress exams is to identify issues with a patient before it gets worse. For instance, you may have a patient who is frustrated with care and they don't verbalize that on their visits but when you give them a subjective feedback form to fill out they finally tell you about their frustrations. You can then address this with them and possibly adapt your plan in order to help them get the best results possible.

Inspire and Train Your Team

The third way that you can use the information gathered during progress exams is to inspire and train your team. Share the subjective feedback forms and objective progress exams with your team during weekly team meetings to remind all of you about the importance of the work that you're doing and the impact you're making in the community.

SECTION 3:
GROWTH MASTERY

"Strength and growth come only through continuous effort and struggle."

-Napoleon Hill

CHAPTER ELEVEN

PLAN YOUR MARKETING FOR GROWTH

The Tools You Need to Develop a Marketing Plan That Works Year after Year

"The best marketing strategy ever: CARE."

– Gary Vaynerchuk

Within the chiropractic community, unfortunately, there is somewhat of a taboo at times when it comes to marketing.

You will hear doctors say things like this:

"I don't do any marketing"

"I just deliver the goods so I don't need to market"

"Results and referrals are all I need"

"I didn't go to school to be a salesman"

This type of mindset within the Upper Cervical Chiropractic Industry is a big reason why 80% of doctors are in solo practice, collecting less than $40,000 per month, and not making a bigger impact in their community.

This anti-marketing mentality is hurting doctors, patients and upper cervical worldwide.

If you look at the top 20% of our great profession (those who are collecting more than $40,000 per month) you will see a consistent pattern of internal and external marketing outreach and a systematized sales process.

These are the doctors who have one or more associates and therefore have freedom, stability, and flexibility in their practice.

119

These top 20% of doctors in the Upper Cervical Field are the ones that we frequently have on our podcast and are being featured in this book. Our goal is to teach you what it takes to grow your practice to the same level.

You may be a doctor that is already in that top 20% which means you are likely someone that is constantly looking for ways to improve and we are confident that you will find this information valuable as well.

UNDERSTANDING THE MARKETING LIFECYCLE

In an interview I did years ago with Dr. Michael Lenarz, even before the podcast, we discussed the importance of understanding the marketing lifecycle of an Upper Cervical Practice.

Whether your practice has been open for a month or 50 years, you are somewhere on the marketing lifecycle.

When you first start in practice and you have no patients your practice must be 100% derived from external marketing outreach.

But over time as your practice builds you should rely less on external marketing outreach and more on internal referral generation with digital marketing integrating them both.

The first 3 to 5 years in practice should be heavily focused on external marketing outreach with somewhere between 60 to 90% of your new patients coming from external sources.

You should reach a turning point somewhere between 3 to 5 years into practice where the majority of your new patients (more than 50%) are coming from internal referral generation.

The tendency when this happens is to become complacent and take your foot off the gas when it comes to external marketing outreach and effectively integrating your digital marketing with both your internal and external strategies. This can be evidence of an arrogance of success happening and can cause your practice to dramatically drop.

Your marketing lifecycle will also depend on your overall goals and how close you are to achieving them. For instance, if you have a goal to have an associate by your fifth year in practice then you want to make sure that you have your marketing in place in order to sustain both you and an associate.

Take into consideration that when you bring on an associate they are most likely starting at zero. That means you will once again have to start at 100% external marketing outreach in the marketing lifecycle in order to generate patients for them.

Your first year in practice you will likely be at 10% internal referral and 90% external marketing outreach. This is the time that you want to be the most aggressive in your community-based marketing and other strategies. When you hit the three to four-year mark your goal should be to attract over 50% of your new patients from referrals and less than 50% should come from external marketing. Over time you should continue to progress to the point where about 90% of your new patients come from referrals and you are not as reliant on external marketing outreach.

The caveat is that I recommend all Upper Cervical Doctors get to the point where they can have at least one associate in their practice. Solo practice is a dangerous game as we discussed earlier. Your goal should be to get to at least $35,000 per month in collections with no more than 50% overhead before you can bring on an associate. If you haven't reached that level yet through your marketing strategy, I recommend continuing to focus on external marketing outreach and digital marketing integration to reach that level so you can bring on an associate and continue to grow.

Once you have established where you are in the marketing lifecycle the next step is to determine your marketing budget in order to achieve your goals.

DETERMINING YOUR MARKETING BUDGET

Frequently when I talk to Upper Cervical Chiropractors about marketing, they are just flying by the seat of their pants.

I frequently hear things like this:

"I really don't have a specific marketing budget."

"I don't actually have a plan in place to reach my goals when it comes to marketing."

"If I have a little bit of extra money this month, maybe I will spend it on marketing"

Most Upper Cervical Practices don't have a marketing director which means that marketing for the practice becomes another responsibility of the clinic director. Some doctors are very skilled at chiropractic marketing, but most struggle in this area, especially when it comes to generating patients from external sources.

Word-of-mouth referrals and internal marketing promotions are excellent ways to maintain the size of your practice. However, if your goal is to increase the size of your practice, you must do some type of external marketing outreach.

The first step in determining what a proper budget would be for your practice when it comes to marketing is to sit down and create SMART goals as we discussed in an earlier chapter. These goals should be specific, measurable, attainable, results focused, and time-dependent goals.

You should have goals for patient visits, new patients, and collections, at the very least.

Next, develop a month by month, week by week and day by day Chiropractic Marketing Plan focused on achieving your goals (more on this later in the chapter).

Once you have figured out the marketing activities that you will be participating in both internally and externally, you can then begin to develop a budget.

A good rule of thumb, based on several sources, is to spend between 2% and 10% of your gross revenue on marketing activities.

For instance, if you collect $30,000 per month you should be spending between $600 and $3,000 per month on marketing, depending on your goals and how aggressively you want to pursue them.

The most successful companies in the world are spending between 7-20% on marketing. Most Fortune 500 companies spend 2% of their annual revenue just on advertising which comes out to be billions of dollars.

The fact is if you want to grow your practice you need to spend some money on marketing.

What you want to look for is a good return on investment. If your case fee is $2000 and you spend $1500 a month on a new marketing program that gets you on average 5 well-educated, prequalified patients per month who all start care, then your $1500 investment just created $10,000 in additional revenue for your practice. Not to mention all of the referrals you're going to generate from those five patients.

That would be an excellent return on investment!

It's important to understand the steps necessary to achieve your goals. For instance, say you want to see 5 more new patients per month for the next six months for a total of 30 new patients. You know that 3 out of every 4 new patients who come into your office start care with you so you determine that you will need to generate 40 new patients from your external marketing over the next 6 month period.

Once you have that information you will need to track backward from 40 new patients to determine how many new patients you need to have per month, per week, and per day that you are in the office. Then establish a chiropractic marketing plan and budget to attract those new patients.

When establishing a budget for your marketing it is essential to consider not only the size of your market but the competitiveness of your market as well. These rules of thumb are a good place to start to determine a marketing budget for Upper Cervical Chiropractors but it is also important to consider the size and competitiveness of your market especially when it comes to digital marketing.

Large Competitive Markets in the US

When it comes to marketing, especially online marketing, it is important to understand the size and competitiveness of the market.

Large competitive markets* include:

- New York City
- Los Angeles
- Chicago
- Houston
- Philadelphia
- Phoenix
- San Antonio
- San Diego
- Dallas
- San Jose

*Based on the 2014 estimates these 10 cities have more than 1 million people in the city alone. This does not include the surrounding areas. If you are in one of these large competitive markets you're likely going to need to spend more on your marketing budget especially for online marketing in order to penetrate a crowded and noisy market.

Another way to evaluate the size of your market for the purpose of determining the competitiveness is to go into the Facebook ads manager and set up a Facebook ad looking at the number of people within a 10-mile radius on Facebook based on the over 30 demographics. If there are more than 500,000 people within a 10-mile radius on Facebook, you are most likely in a large competitive market.

Facebook ads can be extremely powerful, even in a large competitive market, but your budget must be higher in order to compete with all the other advertisers who are going after the same large competitive market.

Online marketing can be highly effective in a large competitive market, but again, you have to have the budget available.

Medium-Sized Markets in the US

We define a medium-sized market as those cities that have between 100,000 and 500,000 people in them within a 10-mile radius on Facebook in the most likely demographic to respond to chiropractic marketing (those over 30). We trim these demographics down by sex, language, age etc. but this is a good place to start when looking at the size of the market.

This would include cities such as:

- Colorado Springs, Colorado
- Lincoln, Nebraska
- St. Louis, Missouri
- Fort Wayne, Indiana
- Omaha, Nebraska
- Wichita, Kansas
- New Orleans, Louisiana
- Reno, Nevada
- Scottsdale, Arizona
- Birmingham, Alabama

There are many other cities that fit this demographic profile.

These medium-sized markets have been some of our most successful locations for running online marketing programs for Upper Cervical Practices.

Small Markets in the US

A small market would be defined as those cities that have less than 100,000 people within a 10-mile radius on Facebook. In these markets, it is not uncommon to be able to draw from a larger distance. We frequently will be able to do successful online marketing programs up to 20 to 25 miles away for Upper Cervical Doctors.

Small markets would include:

- Sioux Falls, South Dakota
- Bentonville, Arkansas
- Montgomery, Alabama
- Evansville, Indiana
- Yarmouth, Maine
- Chambersburg, Pennsylvania
- South Bend, Indiana
- Fargo, North Dakota
- Manchester, New Hampshire
- Billings, Montana

Small markets can be extremely good markets for doing online marketing programs. Typically, with the smallest budget, we can help you make a tremendous impact and dominate your local market.

International Markets

International markets (English-speaking) are completely different than US-based markets. Canada, Australia, Philippines, South Africa, United Kingdom, New Zealand, and other English-speaking nations with Upper Cervical Doctors are wide open for online marketing. We have seen tremendous returns on investment in international markets. If you are in an international market and you are not doing some sort of online marketing then you are missing out on possibly doubling your practice. Within the past year, we have already seen 2 of our doctors double their practices who are in international markets through our online marketing programs alone.

If you would like a tool to help you determine what your marketing budget should be for your Upper Cervical Practice specific to your collections download our complimentary budget calculator resource at www.uppercervicalmarketing.com/budgetcalculator.

THREE ESSENTIALS OF SUCCESS TO ANY UC CHIROPRACTIC MARKETING PLAN

For over 13 years now I have been involved with the marketing of Chiropractic. First as an associate, then as a clinic director, and now as an online marketing agency owner. I have found that there are 3 essentials to the success of any marketing program that you could possibly do for your Upper Cervical Chiropractic Practice.

I believe that if your marketing approach fails for your Upper Cervical Practice it is directly related to one or more of these essentials not being met.

Commitment

The first essential is commitment.

If you are not committed to the marketing approach that you are taking then it will fail or at best it will not work as well as it could if you were committed.

It's not enough to just be involved in the marketing approach that you're doing.

It's like that old saying about ham and eggs:

The chicken was involved, but the pig was committed.

If you are attempting to market your practice in any way make sure you fully commit to the process of succeeding.

Here's one example. If you are a client of ours and are running one of our online marketing programs for your Upper Cervical Practice then we will ask you to get us video testimonials from your practice in order for us to use in your online marketing. We have found that it is an extremely important aspect of social proof to have video testimonials in our system and we use them in a variety of ways.

We will supply you with the questions to ask, make equipment recommendations, and anything else that we know to help you get the best possible video testimonial. However, ultimately, it's your responsibility to get these video testimonials recorded and sent over to us so we can optimize them, promote them, and put them into your system.

We really see a dramatic improvement in conversion and results for our clients when we have these video testimonials in place.

Unfortunately, sometimes we have clients who never get us the video testimonials we ask them for when they first get started with us. Even though we tell them about the importance of video testimonials before we ever launch their program and even when we continue to remind them month after month, some clients just fail to do their part to make their program a complete success.

These are also, unfortunately, usually the doctors who complain about their results and eventually end up canceling their program. They never get to see the full benefit of their complete program in action.

This is just one example of a lack of commitment on the doctor's part resulting in a lack of results with an online marketing approach.

Here's another example that demonstrates a low level of commitment. This example would involve an Upper Cervical doctor who decides to focus on using professional referrals.

Let's say the doctor goes out and meets five different health professionals. Over a six-month period of time they refer 2 people to these five health professionals and at the end of that six months, they say that professional referrals don't work in their area because they never got a referral from any of these health professionals.

This is an example of being involved, but not committed.

To succeed with professional referrals a doctor needs to refer a lot more people to the health professionals that they are working with than they are ever going to get back in return.

The first essential to success is commitment. You must be willing to commit to your marketing approach completely in order to realistically expect a successful outcome.

Strategy

The next aspect of success is the strategy. Once you are fully committed to your marketing approach, you then need to develop a strategy that is going to be effective in executing that approach.

Once again let's use the example of online marketing.

If you are fully committed to blogging for your Upper Cervical Practice and decide to write a blog post for your website one time a week for three months and are expecting to get five new patients per month from your blogging efforts you are going be very disappointed.

Blogging is an important part of a comprehensive online marketing strategy and it is something we do for every single one of our clients but blogging alone is not enough. We have found that blogging is less than 5% of what you need to be doing in order to consistently generate new patients online.

Blogging helps to improve search engine optimization and provides you with content you can share on social media, but as a direct new patient generating strategy it is not very effective.

Even if you execute perfectly on your strategy and you never miss a week of blogging for three straight months, the chances that you will have generated 15 new patients for your Upper Cervical Practice at the end of three months is about zero.

Just because you are committed to a marketing approach does not mean it's going to succeed. You must have the right strategy in place along with the commitment as well as one more essential to guarantee success.

Market

The last essential of success for any marketing approach that you do for your chiropractic practice is your market.

Different markets will have a different response to different marketing approaches.

For instance, some markets may respond extremely well to lunch and learn workshops while other markets may not. Some markets may respond well to business surveys while other markets will not.

The key is to find an effective strategy that has worked in another market and fully commit to it in your market and then see how well it will succeed.

If it does not succeed then it is either your strategy or your market that is the problem. You can attempt to change your strategy and see if you get a better result or move on to a different approach to test in your market.

To use an online marketing example, in some markets such as San Francisco, it is extremely important to get Yelp reviews and it is a major factor in how many new patients you can generate online. But in many small markets across the United States, Yelp is a nonfactor and actually a complete waste of time and money to focus on at all.

This is why it is very important that you connect with other people who understand strategy and market when you are moving into a new marketing approach.

If you want to attract new patients through speaking then find someone else who is doing it effectively and learn from them. If you want to attract new patients from the Internet than talk with us. We have helped upper cervical doctors attract over 20,000 new patients over the past 5+ years and we know what works and what doesn't.

To be successful in any type of marketing for your Upper Cervical Practice you must be fully committed, you must have the right strategy in place, and your market must be receptive to your marketing approach.

CREATING A MARKETING PLAN

Every practice should have a marketing plan for every year.

One of the easiest ways to do this is simply to use our Chiropractic Marketing Plan Calendar. This will allow you to keep track of all your marketing initiatives throughout the year in a digital format that you can also print out and put up on the wall as a daily visual reminder.

You can get the calendar free by going to www.uppercervicalmarketing.com/resources.

Please take a few minutes to go and get this marketing calendar before proceeding with this chapter. I will be referring to it often and it will make more sense if you are able to see the calendar as a reference.

In today's world the most successful Upper Cervical Practices will combine 3 types of marketing in their chiropractic marketing plan:

- Digital Marketing (online marketing)
- External Outreach
- Patient Education and Internal Events

These three types of marketing, when done effectively, will feed into each other and will give you a steady stream of high-quality new patients coming into your office.

This type of marketing strategy will also help you retain the patients you have and reactivate inactive patients.

Digital marketing when done effectively is both an internal marketing approach and an external marketing approach.

Digital marketing should be your first line of both of the boxes on your calendar like this:

January 2019

INTERNAL EVENTS
1. Digital Marketing (newsletter, feedback/online review requests, video testimonials, Doctor videos)
2.
3.

EXTERNAL EVENTS
1. Digital Marketing (Facebook ads, search engine optimization, blogging, social media strategy)
2.
3.

To implement a comprehensive digital marketing program, it can be very complicated and very time-consuming for you or your staff. For the cost of a part-time team member, we can help you implement a comprehensive digital marketing program that will support both your internal and external marketing initiatives.

To learn more, grab a practice health screening for your Upper Cervical Practice at www.uppercervicalmarketing.com.

Once you have your digital marketing figured out, next you want to brainstorm 2 internal events and 2 external events that you will be doing each month. Let's go through some internal events first.

INTERNAL MARKETING

Internal marketing should all be focused on patient education and internal events in some way, shape, or form.

Patient education is the number one way that doctors have been effectively generating new patients internally according to our Upper Cervical Practice Surveys.

You will want to be sure that you have an ongoing patient education strategy for your Upper Cervical Practice.

One of the easiest ways to do this is to get the Upper Cervical Patient Education Station. This is a series of educational flyers that can be used to educate patients on an ongoing basis. Included with this program are 15 UC educational tidbits, 3 patient quizzes, a welcome letter, protocol to implement, and signage art to print out to announce the Education Station program.

This program is very intentional and very effective for creating well-educated patients who will tell others about you and your practice.

You can get this at https://uppercervicalmarketing.com/product/upper-cervical-patient-education-station/

If you decide to implement the education station beginning in January like we would recommend then go ahead and add that to your marketing plan calendar like this.

January 2019

INTERNAL EVENTS
1. Digital Marketing (newsletter, feedback/online review requests, video testimonials, Doctor videos)
2. Education Station Implementation
3.

Another excellent internal marketing promotion to utilize with the

Education Station is the Certificate of Health Program.

The Certificate of Health Program is a way that you can make it easy for your patients to refer others. Anytime you have a patient who mentions a family member, friend or coworker you give them a Certificate of Health which provides that family member, friend or coworker with a discounted first visit with an expiration date.

The Certificate of Health Program is a very effective way to improve your referral conversion as you give someone an incentive and urgency to come in and see you.

We have an entire program on how to effectively do the Certificate of Health Program along with the graphics and implementation you can get in our online store at www.uppercervicalmarketing.com/shop

If you decide this is another initiative that you are going to implement in January go ahead and add it to your internal marketing list like this on your marketing calendar:

January 2019

INTERNAL EVENTS
1. Digital Marketing (newsletter, feedback/online review requests, video testimonials, Doctor videos)
2. Education Station Implementation
3. Certificate of the Health Program Implementation

EXTERNAL MARKETING OUTREACH

Next, you want to decide what 2 external marketing outreach initiatives to begin implementing.

One of the best external marketing outreaches I've seen over the past several years is what's called the Ladies Night of Indulgence.

This outreach program is very effective at attracting more women into your practice. Women are the primary health care decision-makers for their families and it's very important that you attract women into your practice consistently.

If you want to learn exactly how the Ladies Night of Indulgence outreach program works including an implementation protocol, sponsor letter that you can use to solicit other businesses to be involved and personalized flyers that you can use to promote the event, grab our Ladies Night of Indulgence execution plan in our online store at www.uppercervicalmarketing.com/shop.

If you decide to implement this external marketing outreach make sure you are thoroughly promoting this through your online marketing, email and social media formats along with your internal promotion.

If you decide to move forward with this program then go ahead and add that to your list on your marketing plan calendar like this:

EXTERNAL EVENTS
1. Digital Marketing (Facebook ads, search engine optimization, blogging, social media strategy)
2. Ladies Night of Indulgence Event
3.

Another great external marketing outreach initiative to start in January is generating professional referrals from other health practitioners.

We have a ton of great information about generating professional referrals that we will go over in a later chapter.

If you decide to implement a professional referral strategy go ahead and add that to your list like this:

EXTERNAL EVENTS
1. Digital Marketing (Facebook ads, search engine optimization, blogging, social media strategy)
2. Ladies Night of Indulgence Event
3. Professional Referral Strategy

Now you are ready for January with the following marketing plan:

January 2019

INTERNAL EVENTS
1. Digital Marketing (newsletter, feedback/online review requests, video testimonials, Doctor videos)
2. Education Station Implementation
3. Certificate of the Health Program Implementation

EXTERNAL EVENTS

1. Digital Marketing (Facebook ads, search engine optimization, blogging, social media strategy)
2. Ladies Night of Indulgence Event
3. Professional Referral Strategy

Next, you want to add specific dates to the marketing calendar like this:

- Education Station Implementation rollout- Tuesday, January 2
- Certificate of Health Program Implementation rollout- Tuesday, January 2
- Digital Marketing Strategy Session with Upper Cervical Marketing- Wednesday, January 3
- Professional Referral Strategy Implementation- Monday, January 8
- Ladies Night of Indulgence Event- Tuesday, January 23 at 6 PM

Also, you want to add specific dates for support of your initiatives such as:

- Purchase Education Station Materials
- Purchase Certificate of Health Materials
- Purchase Ladies Night of Indulgence Event Implementation Protocol
- Find Five Businesses to Contribute Products or Services to Ladies Night of Indulgence Event
- Promote the Event Via Social Media, Email
- Print Event Flyers Post and Pass out to Patients

NEXT STEPS

Once you lay out a solid plan for success in January, move on to February and March, etc.

You may want to continue certain initiatives that are working well or implement new initiatives such as:

- New Patient Orientation Class
- Dinner with the Doc
- Health Fair Events
- Migraine Headache Case Study Campaign

- Printed Upper Cervical Specific Newsletters
- Report of Findings Booklets
- Upper Cervical Specific Charts and Posters

To find out more about any of these initiatives go to
https://uppercervicalmarketing.com/shop/

INTEGRATING YOUR MARKETING PLAN FOR TODAY'S DIGITAL WORLD

It's time to start thinking differently about how you approach marketing.

Your marketing approaches do not exist in a bubble.

The more effectively you integrate your Chiropractic marketing the better your results will be.

In today's world digital marketing, also known as online marketing or Internet marketing, is the hub between all the other marketing that you do.

Integrating Your New Patient Orientation Class With Facebook Live

For instance, the top Upper Cervical Doctors frequently do a New Patient Orientation Class on a consistent basis. A New Patient Orientation Class a.k.a. a Healthcare Class is one of the most effective ways to build a practice. Helping a new patient understand where true health comes from and how Upper Cervical and specifically your office is equipped to help them reach their health goals is essential for patient compliance, patient education, and creating referrals.

In my professional opinion, every office should be doing a new patient orientation class every 1-4 weeks.

But to get even more benefit from your class and reach both an online and off-line world you can integrate your class online. You will need to make sure that you have at least one CA with you to help you complete the steps below:

The first step is to prepare by getting a tripod and a lapel mic so you have good video and audio. You can get a tripod that integrates well with a smartphone or tablet and a lapel mic through Amazon.

Next, you want to set this up in your lobby or wherever you are doing your class in a place where the camera will see you, any visual aids you are using and your audience if possible.

Once you are set up, you or your CA can open the Facebook app from your phone. Next, go to your business page (make sure you are posting as your business page and not your personal page) and then click on the area that says "write something", then select live video. Write a quick description before going live, maybe something like "Everything You Ever Wanted to Know about Upper Cervical but Were Afraid to Ask" and then start the broadcast as you start your live NPOC for your new patients and guests.

During your broadcast, you'll see the number of viewers, the names of other verified people or Pages who are tuning in, and a real-time stream of comments. Your CA should be logged into Facebook from a PC and monitoring comments and replying as necessary as you do your class.

When you end your broadcast, it will be published on your Timeline so that fans who missed it can watch the video at a later time, although you have the option to remove it just like any other post.

People who like your page can discover your live videos in News Feed and through notifications on Facebook. While watching a live video, people can tap the subscribe button to get notified the next time your page goes live.

This allows you to get a significantly bigger reach for your class. Instead of having 10 people in your class you may have 10 people who are there in person and another 50 who are online during the 30-60 minutes that you're doing your class.

Also, you may have another 50 or more who watch the recording. Depending on the number of fans you have connected to your page this can increase the reach of your class by 10 times and is a tremendous way to integrate your marketing effectively.

Everyone who logs into Facebook during your live class will see your live broadcast near the top of their news feed.

If you do a patient orientation class every week this is a tremendous way to connect with people who are already aware of you to build more trust, credibility, and likability.

Along with this integration strategy, there are many other ways to improve the results of your internal and external marketing strategies by integrating your digital marketing.

Build Your List of Qualified Prospects

There is a digital marketing adage that says: "The money is in the list." This is a true statement IF you know how to build a lead list effectively and nurture the relationships.

The first step to building an effective email list/text list/Facebook message list is to determine your ideal patient profile which we discussed in a previous chapter. If you don't know your ideal patient and how your unique niche serves them then you can't build a list of prospects effectively. Next, you want to put a strategy in place to attract and nurture these leads (we'll talk more about this in a future chapter).

These principles would apply to email follow-up, text-based follow-up via mobile, and also Facebook message follow-up.

Once you have built a list of qualified prospects who:

- are in your local area
- have a condition or demographic profile consistent with your target market
- and have indicated that they want help

Your next step is to invite them to everything that you're doing.

In Michael Port's book, Book Yourself Solid he discusses the concept of always having something to invite people to and this is a great strategy. When you have something to invite people to like a monthly class or a monthly promotion, this will allow you to make a next step offer to the individuals on your prospect lead list.

This can be done both through internal and external promotions. If you're doing a lunch and learn at a particular location, invite everyone on your list to it. If you're having a food drive, invite everyone on your list to it.

You want to send your prospect lead list 3 types of messages:
1. Valuable, educational and actionable information that will help them (this should be the majority of your messages (approximately

75%)

2. Invitations to events both in office and out in the community (approximately 15% of your messages)
3. Direct invitations to schedule a consultation with your office (this should be the smallest percentage of messages approximately 10%)

If you want help building a highly qualified prospect lead list and nurturing that list to produce consistent new patients for years to come schedule a market analysis and blueprint with our team by going to www.uppercervicalmarketing.com.

Integrating Your Internal Marketing Digitally

Here are 3 ways to effectively integrate your internal marketing digitally:

Take Pictures

One of the best ways that you can integrate what you're doing inside your office with the digital world is by taking pictures.

Put one of your CA's in charge of taking pictures every day.

Here is what you want to take pictures of:

- the doctor celebrating with patients who are getting great results
- the team celebrating with patients who are getting great results
- whiteboard selfies are great (write a few lines about the patient's results on a whiteboard and have the patient hold the whiteboard and take a picture with them)
- any events that are going on in the office
- anniversaries
- birthdays

Once you get the pictures send them to your online marketing team or have your marketing CA post them to:

- Facebook
- Instagram
- Pinterest
- Print them out and put them near your jump seat

When you demonstrate through your pictures that your office is a place where people get well and have fun it can be a very powerful way to build trust, credibility, and likability which can improve your referral conversion, retention and new patient generation.

Record Videos

Along with taking pictures, recording videos is another must to thoroughly integrate your internal marketing with the digital world.

Once again have a CA that is designated as a video recorder and give her the goal of recording at least one video per week. If you record one video per week you will capture 52 videos per year which would be tremendous.

Here is what you want videos of:

- video testimonials
- Doctor explanatory videos about upper cervical, specific conditions and frequently asked questions
- the doctor celebrating with patients who are getting great results
- the team celebrating with patients who are getting great results
- any events that are going on in the office

Make sure that if you are going to use your patient's pictures or videos digitally that you have a signed release form from your patient to use their likeness in your marketing. If you need help with this you can get our video testimonial release form as part of our reputation builder toolkit by going to www.uppercervicalmarketing.com/resources.

Once you get the videos send them to your online marketing team or have your marketing CA post them to:

- Facebook
- Instagram (if the video is less than 60 seconds)
- YouTube
- Your Website
- Your lobby TV

Hold Quarterly Contests

Another effective way to integrate what's going on inside your office with the digital world is by holding contests.

Having a quarterly contest where you encourage patients to do helpful tasks both online and off-line for raffle tickets such as:

- New patient referral = 10 tickets
- Video testimonial = 7 tickets
- Google/yelp/Facebook review = 5 tickets
- Facebook check-in = 3 tickets
- Share a Facebook post = 2 tickets
- Like/comment on a Facebook post = 1 ticket

Giveaway something big like a smart TV, tablet, $500 gift card to whole foods or something else that will get someone's attention and make them want to be involved.

You would then want to promote your quarterly contest via social media and through email newsletters to existing patients as well as promoting it in your office.

You also want to take pictures and record videos all along the way to promote the contest as your patients participate and of course when you announce the winner! We will talk more about quarterly contests in the next chapter.

Integrating Your External Marketing Digitally

Upper Cervical Awareness Events

Upper Cervical Awareness Events such as:

- Dinner with the Doctor
- Ladies Night of Indulgence
- Health Topic Classes

These types of events can all be promoted both inside your office, in the community and online.

Inside your office

- Have flyers on every person's chair in the lobby and in every adjusting room.
- Talk with your patients about the event and encourage them to invite others

- Talk to your staff and encourage them to invite others
- Have your staff talk up the event on an ongoing basis

Out in your community

- Pass out flyers to neighborhood businesses
- Post on bulletin boards at Gyms, health food stores etc.
- Talk about the event at your networking groups
- Include an announcement for the event in your email newsletter
- Promote on your social media including Facebook, Instagram, Pinterest with pictures and videos leading up to and at the event

Professional Referral Network Building

Another way to effectively use digital marketing with your external marketing outreach is through your professional referral network building.

If you have other health professionals that refer patients to you give them a shout out on social media:
- Tag their Facebook page and thank them for another referral on your Facebook page
- Recommend their services on your social media (Facebook, Instagram, Pinterest)
- Cross promote events: share events that they are doing and they can promote yours
- Write articles for their website with a link back to yours
- Have them write articles for your website with a link back to their website
- If you have events with multiple health professionals in your office take pictures and videos and post to Facebook, Instagram, YouTube, and Pinterest

Networking Events

Many doctors use networking events to promote their practices and you can make this much more effective by using digital marketing strategies.

If you are involved with a study group, BNI group or another networking group you once again want to take pictures, record short videos, and give shout-outs to other business owners who you recommend.

You can also add business owners that you've met at events to your prospect lead list and invite them to your internal and external events by email, text or Facebook message.

There are many more ways to do this…be creative and have fun with your marketing!

CHAPTER TWELVE

OWN THE 3 R'S OF INTERNAL PRACTICE SUCCESS

Referrals, Retention, and Re-activations

*"There is only one boss. The CUSTOMER.
And he can fire everybody in the company from the
chairman on down, simply by spending his money
somewhere else."*

– Sam Walton

Now that you have an integrated marketing plan for your Upper Cervical Practice, let's get into some specifics and strategies to use both internally and externally.

In this chapter, we are going to discuss the 3R's of internal practice success: referrals, retention, and re-activations.

REFERRALS

Referrals are the lifeblood of any Upper Cervical Practice.

<u>Referrals help maintain your practice while marketing helps your practice grow.</u>

Let's take a look at some ways that the top Upper Cervical Doctors create referrals.

Referral Statements

Dr. Jon Baker coaches some of the top Upper Cervical Doctors in the world and he has a great concept called the referral statement. In episode 28 of the podcast we discussed in detail about referral statements and here are some paraphrased quotes from that podcast about individual visits, progress exams, and group adjusting situations:

Individual Visit

"I've got to make the referral statement...I just finished adjusting you and you get up off the table and you say, "Dr. Baker, I've had more results in your clinic in a week than I've had in 20 years of going to other chiropractors. I'll look you right in the eye and I'll say, "Bill that's not saying bad about them or good about me. This is a very specific office doing specific work, and your body, in this case, requires specific work. I want you to think about this, you've got a wife, you've got three kids, you've got neighbors on each side of you, how many people do you think you know that have no idea about the specific chiropractic we do in this office that might change their life? See your wife may have problems with headaches. She may have problems with her menstrual cycle. She may have no problems yet. Wouldn't you rather have it checked out perfectly and specifically or would you rather wait until you have to drag her in because she can't move?"

Progress Exam

"Let's just say, for example, I'm on a reexamination. You've been under care for 30 days, and I'm very happy with your progress, and I show you on a road to recovery chart where you're at because you need to know. 'Bill you're doing exactly as planned.' One of my concerns would be that if we went and re-X-rayed you today, it wouldn't look any different even though you're feeling great. So, a lot of people that you know think they're feeling great but don't even know that their bodies are decaying and dying inside. You're excited about how you're feeling. Don't just tell people how excited you are about how you're feeling. This week go tell four people exactly what happened when you came to this office for specific chiropractic care."

Group Adjusting

"Mary, do you realize? It's been less than three months since you were referred in this office by Steve, and I remember Steve almost had to drag you into this office. Like a lot of the patients probably in this room laying down laughing right now. But I want you to think about this, what do you think the next 20 years of your life would have been like if you still suffered the way you did the month before you came in here? Mary, this week go out and go on a mission. Go tell five people that you really care about, about specific chiropractic here in this office."

If you and your team are consistently talking with every patient about referrals and using referral statements you will be amazed at how many referrals you can generate.

Increasing Referrals with Books

James Tomasi is an Upper Cervical Chiropractic advocate. His life was literally saved through Upper Cervical Chiropractic care and he wrote a tremendous book called *What Time Tuesday* that can be used as an excellent referral tool.

If you are not familiar with James Tomasi's story, he was suffering from trigeminal neuralgia for years and had lost all hope of recovery. He decided that he was going to escape from the pain by committing suicide. However, on the Tuesday morning that he was planning to commit suicide, he saw an Upper Cervical Chiropractor for the first time and that visit changed the course of his life forever.

It is an amazingly powerful story.

If you have never purchased a case of books from the Tomasi's I highly recommend it.

You can get them here http://whattimetuesday.com/.

The best way that you can utilize books like these to create awareness and ultimately referrals is to just have a commitment from you and your team to give them away to patients.

For instance, if you purchase a case of the *What Time Tuesday* books, you will have about 150 to give away. Set a goal to give away 50 books a week for 3 weeks. You should absolutely see an increase in your referrals, the education of your patients, and the overall passion and excitement that your patients have for Upper Cervical Chiropractic.

Books like James Tomasi's are designed to be both educational and emotionally stirring.

This should be the goal of all your marketing, to connect with both the head and the heart of your patients and potential new patients. I strongly encourage you to get some Upper Cervical Chiropractic related books and spread the word about Upper Cervical Care to your community today!

Increasing Referrals with Quarterly Contests

I mentioned in the last chapter that quarterly contests can be an effective integrated marketing strategy. It is also an excellent way to increase your referrals and referral conversion with social proof.

Social proof including video testimonials on Facebook, YouTube, and your website as well as online reviews on sites like Google, Facebook, Yelp, Health Grades, and Rate MDs are frequently the unseen factor in dramatically increasing your referral conversion.

When someone is considering your office because a friend or family member has recommended you, one of the first things they do in today's digital world is Google you.

This is when your online reputation becomes crucial.

If you have positive social proof it is going to dramatically increase the likelihood of converting someone who was referred to you into someone who is a new patient in your practice.

A quarterly contest is a great way to both increase your referrals now and later by increasing your social proof.

Here's how to do it.

Creating a Quarterly Contest
The first step is to make up your mind to do it and discuss it with your team in order to get them excited about how much fun it's going to be. The energy that you and your team bring to this contest will determine whether or not it is successful.

You want to have several weeks to brainstorm and plan for the launch of the contest. Some of the specific aspects of the contest to brainstorm with your team include:

- Prize or prizes
- Giveaways
- Raffle or Different Type of Contest

- Activities and Rewards Associated
- Ways to Promote Internally
- Ways to Promote Externally
- Ways to Promote Digitally
- Theme
- Who Is Responsible for What?

One of the really fun parts of doing a quarterly contest is having a grand prize and several other smaller prizes for the winners of the contest. If your contest has a theme you can try to unite your prizes with your theme or you can just give away some big-ticket items that you believe your patients would be excited to win.

Here are some ideas:

- Three or Four Day Cruise for Two
- A Weekend at a Bed and Breakfast
- Platinum TV
- iPad
- Year-Long Gym Membership
- Three Months of Free Groceries from a Natural Grocery Store
- Tickets to a Concert
- Tickets to a Sporting Event
- Movie Tickets
- Restaurant Gift Cards
- Health Food Store Gift Cards
- Custom Pillow
- Books

Whether you choose just one grand prize or a grand prize with a few smaller prizes the key is choosing prizes that your patients would be excited about and you and your team will know that better than anyone else.

Giveaways

Along with raffle prizes you may also want to have some giveaways during the contest. These can help keep people engaged for the full three months you are running the contest. This could be a weekly giveaway for a free massage, free adjustments or a bottle of supplements. The key again is to give something that is exciting and fun to your patients. You would frequently give this to the patient who accumulated the most raffle tickets that week.

Raffle and Rewards

A raffle is usually the best format for this type of quarterly contest. All you need is a roll of raffle tickets and a large glass container to keep the tickets in at your front desk. It is important to have this visual in order to continue to remind people about the quarterly contest each time they are in your office. You should display your prizes in a prominent location in your office to keep the excitement going. Have a system in place that assigns a specific amount of raffle tickets for different activities that patients can do during the quarter.

For instance:

- 10 Tickets = Referral of Friend or Family Member
- 8 Tickets = Bringing a Friend to a Class
- 7 Tickets = Video Testimonial
- 5 Tickets = Google Review
- 4 Tickets = Facebook, Yelp, Health Grades, or Rate MDs Review
- 3 Tickets = Facebook Check-In
- 2 Tickets = Sharing a Facebook Post
- 1 Ticket = Liking Our Facebook Page

Ways to Promote Internally

To promote this event internally you will want to create some key pieces of promotional material including:

- Posters
- Flyers
- Postcards
- Signs

You want to make sure that everyone in your practice knows that this contest is happening. This means that you and your team should be talking consistently about the contest with every patient on every visit.

You should also have posters, counter and table signs and flyers around the practice with information about the contest, prizes and the ways to accumulate raffle tickets.

You can also send out a mailing to your patients with a postcard describing the contest.

Ways to Promote Externally

Although this is primarily an internal promotional event you can certainly promote it externally as well including putting up posters on local bulletin boards or talking about this during community events you might be doing such as talks, screenings, etc.

Ways to Promote Digitally

Digital promotion can be very effective for a quarterly contest. You can send out a series of email blasts about once every other week for the first six weeks and then once a week for the second five weeks. The last week before the raffle drawing send three email blasts encouraging your patients to get as many raffle tickets as possible before the big grand prize is given away. You would want to do a similar type of posting schedule to Facebook utilizing a flyer type picture that you can consistently post promoting the event on Facebook and other social networks such as Instagram, Pinterest, etc.

If you do a consistent monthly email newsletter, and we highly recommend that you do, you would also want to promote the contest within your newsletter every month during the quarter.

Theme

Some doctors like to have a theme for each quarter and have their contest correspond with their theme.

For instance, some themes that doctors have done successfully include:

- Nutrition
- Fitness
- Stress Management
- Condition Specific: Multiple Sclerosis, Migraines, Alzheimer's, Parkinson's Etc.

If you choose to do a theme then you can have all of your giveaways and prizes focused around that particular theme. You might also want to have events that are scheduled throughout the quarter related to that theme including in-office classes, walks or other events related to specific conditions. Just one example would be having your team and your patients participate in a Memory Walk for Alzheimer's.

Who Is Responsible for What?

The last and most important aspect of doing a fantastic quarterly contest is to have different members of your team take ownership of different aspects of the contest. Once you have brainstormed and laid out a plan for the contest each member of your team should have different responsibilities in order to execute the plan.

Some offices will do quarterly contests every quarter of the year while others may choose to only do a big giveaway once a year. If you have never done a quarterly contest, I highly recommend you plan and execute one to see how your practice responds. It just might be a game changer for you and your practice when it comes to increasing your referrals and social proof which will have an impact on your practice for years to come.

RETENTION

Along with generating referrals, the second "R" associated with internal practice success is retention. It is much more cost effective to keep a patient than it is to get a new patient.

One of the easiest techniques you can use in order to improve your retention is future pacing.

Future Pacing

Future pacing is the art of always letting your patients know what to expect and what is coming.

A great way to use future pacing is to let patients know about their upcoming progress exam.

"Mary, I know this is only your 4th visit, but remember I told you we are going to re-examine you on your 12th visit. Progress exams are exciting visits for our patients as they get to see and realize their amazing results. I can't wait to see yours!"

Another opportune time to use future pacing is when discussing wellness care.

"Peter, you may already be wondering how you are going to maintain your results after we are done with the structural component of your care. Don't worry, at that point, we will talk about a wellness plan that will have you coming in for maintenance visits that we will schedule according to your needs. We want to sustain these results for a lifetime!"

Feel free to use this technique whenever you feel appropriate. At times, you may get the feeling that patients are already looking for the exit sign because they feel so much better.

Here is another beauty in that situation:

"Jim, you have been doing well with your care and it is evident you are feeling much better. Remember that pain is just the tip of the iceberg and the cause we need to correct is the bigger part of the iceberg that lies below the surface. This is why we do objective progress exams so you don't have to judge your health by how you feel. Yours is coming up in 10 visits! I can't wait to see your results."

By future pacing your patients, you take control of their results. We all know the miracle stories happen after the pain is gone, so higher retention means more amazing stories, more referrals, and a booming practice.

Remember that patients need to be led. It is your responsibility to be their Doctor and lead them through future pacing all the way to wellness care.

Retention Marketing

Retention marketing is focused on keeping your patients. On a daily, weekly, and monthly basis your team should be focusing on retention-based marketing.

Here are 3 excellent ways that you can do retention marketing:

Progress Exams

As we discussed in chapter 10, progress exams are essential to the success of top Upper Cervical Doctors. Progress exams are also one of the best ways that you can retain your patients. By consistently doing a progress exam with your patients every 10 to 12 visits you will keep them engaged in their healing process and their overall progress. Patients forget how unhealthy they were when they started care. Progress exams help them to take a realistic look at how far they've come and is a great opportunity for you to remind them of the potential for continuing care. The combination of the subjective and the objective during the progress exam can be a very powerful combination in promoting patient retention and referrals.

Teach to Testify

When your patients begin to get results it is important that you help them put that into words so they can tell others their story. One of the best ways that you can do this is by having them complete an online review. This will help them to organize their thoughts about what has taken place in their body since they began care, while at the same time improving your ability to attract more patients from the Internet. Another way that you can teach them to testify is by having them do a video testimonial. Once again this will highlight in their mind how far they have come while helping you reach more people online by the distribution and promotion of that video testimonial. We will talk more about the importance of social proof in a future chapter.

Monthly Email Newsletters

Monthly email newsletters are an excellent way to promote patient loyalty, patient compliance, patient retention, online reviews, and referrals. Keeping Upper Cervical and your office at the forefront of your patient's mind is extremely important in today's chaotic world. People forget. They forget why they came to see you originally, they forget what it is you do, and they forget how much progress they've made. Monthly email newsletters are a great way to continue to educate and remind your patients about the long-term benefits of Upper Cervical Care.

Internal Marketing Approaches to Promote Retention and Referrals

Along with the retention marketing strategies we mentioned previously, another way to promote retention and referrals is by consistently doing these essential internal marketing approaches.

Healthcare Classes

Earlier in the book we talked about how Dr. Corinne Weaver has used classes including healthcare classes to grow her practice.

Healthcare classes, also called new new patient orientation classes, are an terrific way to...

- educate new patients
- improve patient compliance, loyalty, retention, and results
- promote referrals

You have 3 main options when it comes to healthcare classes...

1. Do the healthcare class yourself weekly, biweekly or monthly
2. Have an Associate do the class
3. Have a professional New Patient DVD created.

The Pros and Cons of Doing Healthcare Classes Yourself

Pros:
- Helps remind you of why you do what you do
- You can develop a stronger relationship with the patients that attend the class
- If you are a strong speaker and closer you are able to promote more referrals

Cons:
- Time and energy away from your family
- Patients don't always show up
- Spouses and other guests don't always show up
- Classes are not consistent: some classes are better than others

The Pros and Cons of Having an Associate Do Your Class

Pros:
- Frees you up to spend more time with your family
- Teaches your associate to communicate, speak in public, etc.

Cons:
- They may not bring the passion and focus that you bring
- Patients don't always show up
- Spouses and other guests don't always show up
- Classes are not consistent: some classes are better than others

The Pros and Cons of Professionally Created New Patient DVD's

Pros:
- Frees you up to spend more time with your family
- Allows patients, spouses, and families to watch the DVD at home and at their convenience
- The DVD can be given to a friend, family member, or coworker interested in Upper Cervical
- Existing patients can also utilize the DVD to refer others to your practice
- Consistent, clear, and focused message delivered to your patients and potential patients every time

Cons:

- Not all patients will watch the DVD (If you emphasize that watching the DVD or attending the class will help them to get faster results you will have a higher compliance rate.)
- Initial creation cost

If you would like to learn more about the New Patient DVD Program go to https://uppercervicalmarketing.com/new-patient-dvd/.

Internal Events
Along with healthcare classes, internal events are some of the most consistent new patient producers of all internal marketing approaches.

Here's a list of some of the most effective internal events that Upper Cervical Practices can utilize throughout the year.

Patient Appreciation Days (PAD)
Patient Appreciation Days is a great way to promote patient loyalty while increasing referrals. A good time to do this event is on your practice's anniversary. A typical way to do it is to provide complimentary office visits for your regular practice members on one day of the week and complimentary new patient visits on another day of the week. Frequently this type of event is combined with a food drive, toy drive, backpack drive etc.

Food Drives
Thanksgiving and Easter are good times of year for these events. Collect non-perishable food items in exchange for an office visit for an existing patient or a new patient service such as an exam.

Toy Drives at Christmas
Your office can become a Toys-for-Tots drop-off during the Christmas holiday season. Once again you can provide office visits and new patient services in exchange for toys. These types of events promote goodwill in the community, patient loyalty and promote referrals.

Backpack Drives in July and August for Back to School
A backpack drive is another way to do this type of internal promotion event. You can have existing and new patients bring in a new backpack full of school supplies and donate them to a school in your area in exchange for office visits and new patient exams.

Holiday Specials

Some doctors have found good results by having Valentine's Day, St. Patrick's Day, Memorial Day, Labor Day, Veterans Day, etc. specials to promote referrals. These events don't require you to give services away if you don't want to, you can simply offer a discounted price. Some doctors do choose to give away office visits, new patient exams, and x-rays but it is up to the individual doctor to make that decision.

Referral Certificates

As we discussed in the previous chapter a certificate of health type referral certificate program is a great internal marketing strategy to generate more referrals of your patient's friends and family members.

Here is a more detailed explanation on how to do this effectively in your office:

Dr: Mrs. Jones it is fantastic that you are getting such great results with your migraines

Mrs. Jones: Yes, it is just absolutely incredible!

Dr: I bet you have been bragging to your friends and family about how much better you have been doing since you came to our office.

Mrs. Jones: Well I have been talking to my neighbor, Mrs. Smith across the street who also gets migraines.

Dr: Wow, has Mrs. Smith been getting migraines for as long as you have?

Mrs. Jones: No, she actually has been getting them even longer than I have!

Dr: Well that's not good! Mrs. Jones, if I give you something for Mrs. Smith to come in and see if we can help her the way that we have been able to help you, do you promise to give it to her?

Mrs. Jones: Absolutely

Dr: I'm going to give you a special certificate that we only give to our patients for their friends and family. It will allow Mrs. Smith to be able to come in and find out if we can help her with her migraines like we've helped you. Does that sound good?

Mrs. Jones: Yes

Dr: Okay, let's go up to the front desk and have Linda put together a special certificate for Mrs. Smith.

Then, when you get up to the front desk talk to your front desk person about the promise that Mrs. Jones has made to give the referral certificate to her neighbor.

I recommend creating these certificates on nice paper that the patient will handle more gently (you can also get the certificate of health program from our store). The certificate can be for a free consultation, exam, and x-rays or a discounted fee for any or all of these services. The idea is to make the offer attractive enough to get Mrs. Smith into your office.

Monthly Holding Is Healing Contest

Another fun way to promote retention and ingrain our basic Upper Cervical Philosophy in the mind of your patients is to have a Holding Is Healing Contest each month.

In my practice, we would love when patients were holding their adjustment because we knew that they were healing. So we celebrated it by giving patients high-fives, cheering, and being excited for them. We also would reward them for taking such good care of their spine and nervous system in between visits with a raffle ticket every time they held their adjustment.

Then at the end of the month, we would draw one of the tickets from the Holding Is Healing Jar that we kept at the front desk checkout area and give away something fun like an hour massage or a gift certificate to Trader Joe's or another healthier grocery store. Try this. Your patients will love it and so will your team and it's a great way to improve retention.

RE-ACTIVATIONS

The third and final "R" associated with internal practice success is re-activations. No matter how good your practice is there are going to be patients who fall off the map. This might happen if they go on a vacation and never get back on track with care after they return or if they move away for a while and are now back in the area or maybe they just felt so much better that they didn't feel like they needed to continue care. Whatever the reason may be, there will be certain individuals who will not continue with care and it is important that you have strategies in place to reactivate these inactive patients.

156

One of the most important ways to reactivate old patients is by having consistent workshops and other events that you can invite people to. If you consistently have events planned throughout the year, you can reactivate old patients by inviting them to your events.

Monthly email newsletters and social media posts can help with re-activations by keeping you in the forefront of your inactive patient's minds. Make sure you collect email addresses from all of your patients and consistently send them a monthly email newsletter that is relevant to their health and provides good information.

Another excellent way to reactivate old patients is through our 5 Star Doc Reputation Management System. Utilizing your email list, we send a feedback first email to your patients asking for their feedback on your clinic.

Positive feedback is redirected to your online review sites. This system not only generates online reviews (5 – 10 per month on average) but it is also great at creating re-activations.

If the patient had great results in your office and just has stopped coming in for whatever reason, a reminder of the great results that they had by giving you feedback is frequently the nudge they need to schedule an appointment.

Recently one of our doctors had 2 re-activations in the first 3 days of running our 5 Star Doc System.

This system will also give you a good understanding of how satisfied your patients are with your services. Our system automatically gives your practice a Net Promoter Score (NPS) which is a cumulative score based on the feedback received from your patients. This net promoter score is a good indication of how likely your patients are to refer others.

To learn more about the 5 Star Doc Reputation Management System go to www.uppercervicalmarketing.com. You can get this individually or as part of our full digital marketing system. An inactive patient is simply an active patient waiting for the right motivation to change their status.

CHAPTER THIRTEEN

BUILD A POSITIVE PRACTICE REPUTATION

The Power of Social Proof

"It's ironic how fortune disappears once reputation and character is damaged."

– Jon Michail

To be successful in today's digital world your Upper Cervical Practice must have a positive reputation. Your online reputation will make a tremendous difference in how many new patients you generate and how effectively you convert referrals.

CREATING A CULTURE OF SOCIAL PROOF

In his book, *Influence*, psychologist Robert Cialdini discusses the power of social proof. He points out that we rely on others, especially in foreign environments or environments that we are not confident in, to make decisions.

For instance, when someone is considering going to an Upper Cervical Practice for the first time, this is a foreign environment for them. Due to the foreign nature of the situation and with no established confidence, the individual will rely heavily on social proof. The experience of others will be extremely important to their decision-making.

Relatable people to this individual will have an even greater impact on their decision-making.

For instance, if a 45-year-old Caucasian woman with migraines was considering coming into your practice then someone else who is a migraine sufferer and is of a similar age and race will have a strong influence on that person.

If you are looking to attract more athletes to your practice then having social proof that utilized athletes would be most effective. If you would like to attract more pregnant patients, then have social proof that utilizes other pregnant women.

Here are some more examples of the similarity principle in action to connect with your ideal patient profile:

- Women for Women
- Men for Men
- Condition for Condition
- fibromyalgia for fibromyalgia
- Ethnicity for Ethnicity
- Filipinos in the Philippines
- Occupation for Occupation
- office workers for office workers
- Life Situation for Life Situation
- Example Pregnant Women
- Example Mothers Whose Sons Play Hockey

Examples of Social Proof

Two of the most powerful forms of social proof when it comes to online marketing are online reviews and video testimonials. When you use the principle of similarity and social proof together in your online reviews and video testimonials it can be a winning combination.

Online Reviews

Online reviews are critical to your Upper Cervical Practice. Nearly every one of your new patients has read your online reviews (93%).

Here are just some of the statistics from a 2017 Online Review Survey from Bright Local:

- **85% of consumers trust online reviews as much as personal recommendations**
- 93% of consumers read online reviews

- Star rating is #1 factor used by consumers to judge a business
- The average consumer expects to see 34 reviews before feeling able to trust the accuracy of a business' star rating
- 77% of consumers believe reviews older than 3 months are not relevant anymore and don't consider these in their decision making.

So the take-home point is that people today trust online reviews as much as a personal recommendation (that's a referral, folks).

This is huge. This means that if people read enough reviews they trust you as much as if their neighbor told them about you.

Other things to keep in mind when it comes to reviews include:

- You can never have too many (the average person begins to trust the businesses star rating at 34 reviews)
- in a small market, you should have at least 25 reviews on Google
- in a medium-size market, you should have at least 50 reviews on Google
- in a large competitive market, you should have at least 100 reviews on Google
- another good rule of thumb is to have twice as many reviews as anyone else in your city
- Star rating is the number one factor when it comes to reviews.
- You should have at least a 4 ½ out of five-star rating.
- You can't just get a bunch of reviews and then stop. Reviews older than three months are not relevant to most people.
- The best practice is to consistently get reviews every month

Where should you get reviews?

Google is the most important place to have reviews. In every market, Google is an important factor in online marketing success. It is essential that you establish a culture in your practice where you consistently get Google as well as other reviews.

Some other sites that you might want to get online reviews for (depending on your market) are:
- Yelp
- Facebook
- HealthGrades
- Rate MDs

160

If you want to know which sites are the most important for your area, Google your name (Dr. John Smith Dallas Texas) and your practice name (Smith Chiropractic Dallas Texas) to see which review sites come up on the first page of the search results.

How do you get online reviews consistently?
Online reviews have been around for over 10 years. However, most Upper Cervical Chiropractic Practices have less than 10 Google reviews and many doctors have no reviews at all.

The most common reasons why people don't get online reviews for their practice are that they:

- don't know that it's important
- have not made it a priority
- have tried but patients forget as soon as they leave their office

Review handouts and other tools can be useful in showing people step-by-step instructions on how to leave you reviews. Even with this information in hand, unfortunately, many patients will simply not take the time to leave you a review.

Another strategy is sending out emails to all your patients in an attempt to get reviews. While this strategy will most likely result in reviews, you could end up with some negative reviews that bring down your star rating. There was a change to Google's terms of service in 2018 that made all review generators unable to filter out negative feedback so it's very important that if you send out an email blast or use a review generator like ours that you thoroughly clean your list of any emails that may leave you a negative review.

To find out more about our 5 star Doc Reputation Management System go to www.uppercervicalmarketing.com.

Along with our automated review generator here are some other tips to get all of your raving fans on to Google to give you a review. The people from your practice that you ideally want to review you should have these 3 things in common:

1. They have had a great experience in your practice
2. They have a Google account or are willing to create one
3. They will take the time to actually create the review

When collecting Google reviews it's always nice to start with the low hanging fruit. And these are the individuals that already have Google/Gmail accounts.

If your patient management software has the ability to search by email or sort by email and you can determine which of your existing patients have Gmail accounts which is a great way to get started. If not, you will need to put all of your patients into an Excel document and then sort by Gmail addresses.

Next, go through these steps:

1. Have your CA give you a list of existing patients with Gmail accounts
2. Go through the list and highlight the ones that you know have had a great experience
3. Coordinate with your staff when those individuals are going to be in the practice next
4. Go through the process of leaving a review through your smartphone with your staff so that everyone knows how to do it with a Google account
5. Ask these individuals to take a few minutes before they leave today and leave you a review on Google.

Depending on the size of your practice and the size of your list you may be able to get close to 25 Google reviews just from patients with Gmail accounts.

Once you have gone through all of your Gmail addresses, next you want to identify patients who have had a great experience in your practice and request a review from them.

Many patients who are raving fans will be willing to create a Google account if necessary to give you a review. These patients are usually happy to help spread the word about what you are doing in your office to the rest of the community if you properly frame the request.

Lastly, you can ask friends and family to leave you reviews, they are some of your best supporters.

Again, an easy way to do all of this automatically is by using our 5 Star Doc Automated Review Generator. This program uses a feedback first approach to automatically find your raving fans and direct them to Google to leave you a great review and it walks them through the process step-by-step.

Remember people will continue to look for doctors like you online and online reputation will become more and more important.

Some notes on Yelp

As I mentioned previously in this chapter in some markets, especially large competitive markets, Yelp can be a very important factor in generating new patients online and for your referral conversion.

However, some of the most sensational reviews of your services from your actual patients may be ignored or discredited by Yelp. Yelp uses an algorithm which determines the credibility of any review posted on its site, and it also filters for the information that it believes will be "the most helpful and useful to our audience of consumers."

Unfortunately, the ways that Yelp filters reviews can negatively impact your online reputation, even if unintentionally.

That's why it's important to understand how the Yelp review filtering process works. By understanding how Yelp rates your reviews, you can make meaningful changes to your online reputation management tools.

1) Why would my review be filtered?

Some doctors and other business owners believe that Yelp purposefully features negative reviews while filtering out positive ones, however, Yelp insists that the Yelp filtering software looks for specific warning signs that would render a review worthy of filtration. These warning signs can help you if you're trying to create an effective online reputation management campaign.

These warning signs include:

- Multiple reviews from the same IP address, because this suggests that the business owner asked for reviews at their place of business (a practice that Yelp dislikes)
- Unhelpful rants or raves about a place of business

According to Yelp, only 25% of submitted reviews are filtered off the site, so if you feel like your patients have been unduly censored, contact Yelp customer support to express your concern.

2) Filtered reviews vs "other reviews that are not currently recommended"

Yelp used to remove reviews that they did not want to prominently show to their website visitors. Yelp now shows those reviews as "other reviews that are not currently recommended."

So what makes Yelp want to promote some reviews and choose not to recommend others?

One reason that Yelp might choose to treat one review differently than another could be because of the person posting the review because Yelp favors people who post detailed reviews for multiple businesses listed on their website.

3) Expert perspective from elite opinion

Individuals who post many reviews on Yelp are considered elite contributors to the service. Yelp elite members are selected by Yelp itself and are given high marks for a variety of details pertaining to their reviews including:

- The authenticity of the reviewer, as certified through the detail in their opinions and the information included on their profile
- The variety of the contributions to Yelp, as exemplified by the diversity of services that they leave reviews for on Yelp
- The degree of social interaction which the reviewer engages in on the service, which will depend on whether they favor other reviews and on how they contribute to Yelp forums

Yelp elite candidates are also interviewed by Yelp itself because Yelp wants to be sure that its candidates are effective representatives of the services that Yelp offers. Having a positive review from a Yelp elite member means that you will have a positive review that is likely to remain unfiltered.

Although you cannot control what people say about you on Yelp, or how Yelp filters your reviews, knowing what types of reviews are often filtered and which ones are featured can only help as you consider your Yelp profile.

When potential patients are looking for your practice online, your Yelp profile will potentially be one of the first things that they look at especially if you are in a large competitive market. That's why it's important to try and obtain positive reviews from Elite Yelpers and to work with Yelp if you believe your reviews have been unfairly censored.

Video Testimonials

Video testimonials are another excellent way to use the principle of social proof and similarity to improve the results of your online marketing.

When capturing video testimonials, it is important to focus on the emotion behind the condition. People watching the video who are struggling with the same health condition will understand what the person in the video is going through. As they watch, they will begin to imagine what their life would be like if they weren't struggling with their health anymore. This is called the before and after state of the person.

To connect with the before-and-after state of a person, here are some key questions to ask:

1) *What is your first name and where are you from?*

You want the people watching to be able to relate to the individual in the video. Hearing them say their name and where they are from helps the person watching connect with them. It can also be good for optimization and similarity.

2) *What was your life like before coming to our office?*

This question connects with the individuals watching it because they will hear similar feelings, limitations, treatments, results etc. that they are currently experiencing.

3) *What is your life like now?*

This is crucial. When a patient expresses the dramatic difference that Upper Cervical Care has made in their life they can help push a potential new patient to seek the help they need.

4) *How do you see your life going forward now that you have been helped?*

This question basically wraps it all together and helps the individual watching to see what is possible for them in the future if they seek care in your office.

How do you capture video testimonials?

I have seen extremely effective video testimonials done by both professional videographers and by amateurs using an iPhone. I do not believe that it is necessary to hire a videographer in most cases.

The most important aspect of getting a good video testimonial is to make sure people can clearly see the person that is speaking. To accomplish this, you will need a tripod for the device that you are utilizing. Whether you are using an iPhone, an iPad, or a video camera the most important thing is to make sure the video is not shaky.

The 2nd most important part is that you can hear them clearly. You can get a lapel mic or a mic that connects to an iPad to help improve your audio. Get both of these items for less than $100 total on Amazon.

Do you need to get permission to use a video testimonial?

Once you have a video testimonial that looks and sounds fantastic, you need to be sure to get permission to be able to use the video testimonial in your marketing. Make sure you have a video testimonial release form signed by each patient which states that you can use their video in your marketing.

You can have fantastic video testimonials and not be successful in online marketing because you do not have a comprehensive program in place to utilize those video testimonials effectively in all aspects of your marketing.

Video testimonials can be used on your website, social media, landing pages, Facebook ads, email autoresponders, blog posts, email newsletters etc.

You can never have too many online reviews or video testimonials.

Creating a culture of social proof in your office where you are continually discussing the importance of gathering online reviews and video testimonials with your team and your patients will pay off now and for years to come.

CHAPTER FOURTEEN

GROW THROUGH PROFESSIONAL REFERRALS

Win-Win-Win Relationships with Health Practitioners

"Nothing influences people more than the recommendation of a trusted friend."

– Mark Zuckerberg

Another fantastic way to build a practice is through professional referrals. Professional referrals are generally when other health practitioners refer patients to you.

These health care providers would be people you respect and agree with on their approaches to patient care.

They are practitioners that you would trust to take good care of your patients.

It is a win-win-win relationship for everyone, the practitioner, the patient, and you.

It benefits your patients because they are getting better overall care. It is to your benefit because when you refer a patient to another practitioner that does a good job, you look good and it is good for your reputation. It also benefits the other practitioner because they are receiving more referrals as well.

But if you go into it with a shortcut mentality where you say "I referred 3 people to this person and they have not referred anyone to me!" Your heart is not in the right place.

PROFESSIONAL REFERRALS FROM
AN INDIVIDUAL PRACTITIONER

Over the years I have interviewed many doctors who had great success with professional referral relationships including Dr. Jeff Scholten. Dr. Jeff generates 60% of his new patients from professional referrals in a million-dollar practice. In 2014 we had an extensive conversation about professional referrals in which Dr. Jeff shared some great information that we then published in a series of blog posts.

In the sections below I'm going to share a variety of paraphrased quotes from that interview to give you a great foundation on how to build a practice through professional referrals.

Dr. Jeff Scholten: "What is interesting is when you look at the different techniques; a lot of them try to do everything for everybody. But in Upper Cervical Chiropractic we have this challenge and simultaneous opportunity which is that the likelihood of us helping somebody is very high but we really don't know whether the cause of the issue is the subluxation in the upper cervical spine. And the only way to really know is to take care of the subluxation and see what happens to the person's health."

Dr. Scholten continues "We limit our practice and we recognize simultaneously that there are other aspects of health that influence people's ability to hold the reduction or correction that we make. We want our patients to hold (their adjustment), we want them to stabilize, and we want them to recover, so building a referral network is just logical.

I went on a journey of trying to understand what other practitioners are doing so I could understand when it might be appropriate for me to refer a patient to another practitioner. In that process of finding out what other practitioners are doing, they would inevitably start asking what I do for patients."

Dr. Scholten continues "There is really no gimmick here at all. It is just a normal personal relationship. You look, you find people that you like authentically, that you respect professionally, and that you think your patient's personality meshes with. Then you refer your patient to the practitioner that fits their need and who can properly treat them.

It is just about trying to help people on their journey towards optimizing their own personal health.

Along the way, I have met a lot of different practitioners and many of them have ended up sending patients my way. That has turned out to be a wonderful and sustainable way for me to have a practice, and it continues to this day as I continue to meet new people." Dr. Scholten said.

"For example, I went to a physio clinic last night that opened on the 5th floor of our building. I was speaking with the physios and the physician interns trying to understand what they do and thinking about who I might be able to send to them. This resulted in them asking me what I do and who they might be able to send to me. That is the way it works.

Professional referrals are not really that hard to get. I think a lot of people try to shortcut it and forget that it is a relationship like any other. You have to be authentic in that relationship and in your inquisitive nature. If you don't really care and you don't really want to know but you just want to get the benefits, you are probably not going to be successful with it." Dr. Scholten said.

You have to be professional to get a professional referral.

Dr. Scholten continues "When a person puts their reputation on the line and sends somebody to you, you have to really understand the depth of what that means. They are saying, "This is the person that I think can help you", and they are sending that person to you, and you have to steward that appropriately. You have to make sure that the person has a great experience.

If you take spectacular care of them and add that plus one level of service so that they go back to the referring practitioner and say, "Thank you for that referral. That was very helpful. I really appreciate it." Even if they choose not to start care, if they can tell the practitioner that referred them, "I had a great experience but I chose not to start." That's still a win."

The number one thing that you can do wrong is to mess up the first referral from any practitioner.

Dr. Scholten continues "Health practitioners talk to each other, so if you mess up that first referral from someone, it's going to come back to bite you.

I get referrals from physicians and dentists that I have never met and I have never personally talked to. They refer patients to me because they heard from another health practitioner that I might be a person that they would want to refer to. The first step in getting a professional referral is being professional in how you deal with your clinic and being patient-centric. It has to be able to help the patient. **It is not about us. It is about the patient.** ”

Summary Points about Professional Referrals from Individual Health Practitioners

- You need to have the right mindset and the right heart that is focused on the good of the patient to be successful at professional referral relationships
- You will need to go into the community and develop relationships with other health practitioners by calling their offices, visiting their practices, and learning about what they do and how best you can help your patients by referring people to them
- You will need to refer many more patients to other health practitioners than you will receive back from them (it's never a one for one)
- Once you develop a solid network of health professionals in your community you can get consistent new patient referrals from a variety of sources every month

BUILDING AN INTEGRATED COMMUNITY OF HEALTH PROFESSIONALS

Another excellent way to develop professional referral relationships is by building an integrated community in your area. Dr. Giancarlo Licata has a tremendous referral network of several hundred practitioners in his community in the Pasadena California area where he is able to generate about 80% of his new patients from his professional referral network.

In episode 40 of the podcast, we discussed in detail how he has built this community and what he does to nurture relationships that are for the good of the patient.

Here are some paraphrased quotes from that interview:

Dr. Giancarlo Licata: “It's important that you are able to host 10-15 health practitioners in your front lobby for your first meeting. Write a list of ten health practitioners in your community that you want to meet, and then go out and start meeting them. Introduce yourself, and get a feel for them, ask yourself does this person really want to interact with me? It has to start with a relationship and then you can begin to tentatively plan with them and set expectations."

Dr. Licata continues "I say something like...

"We're doing a study group. It's a way for us to build relationships, but it's not networking. Networking is like, stepping into a pool of piranhas. Everybody wants to eat each other and nobody wants to give. Everybody wants to take. This is going to be designed for collaboration. It's going to be designed on relationship building that's longer-term and it's going to be built upon creativity. It will be the first Tuesday of the month at 7 PM at my office, would you be interested in coming."

There is going to be certain people that are going to resonate with that.

There are some others that just don't have the time or energy for it."

Dr. Licata continues "Begin with your first 10, and then look for 10 more for that next month. This will help create enough diversity, enough of a pool of people that are going to come in and out through the seasons but are all going to stay connected, and so, now after years, we have a database of well over 100 practitioners that we have amazing relationships with.

I also try to refer to the health practitioners that attend right away. I keep them at the top of my mind during that month in case there is a genuine opportunity for a referral and there's a need for a patient. So, that way that person is getting some referrals and they're willing to keep investing their time and energy."

Dr. Licata continues "I decided to limit the group to clinical health issues and topics but you can do whatever you want to do. You also want to get feedback from the practitioners who attend and then you can make changes for month three, four, five and six. It's important to understand that you're playing the long game. Don't be upset when you don't get a referral off of that first meeting. Also, this is not a BNI style group where you only have one practitioner from each discipline."

Dr. Licata continues "We have many physical therapists, chiropractors, dentists etc. and that diversity is very valuable because people are going to be attracted to different types of people.

171

For instance, we have close to 10 acupuncturists in our group right now and I naturally gravitate towards two of them. I just really get along with them. We see things the same way, and it doesn't mean that I don't refer to the others, but I'm going to refer more to them just based on personality, trust, and a level of excellence that we both share."

Summary Points about Building an Integrated Community of Health Professionals

- You need to have the right mindset and the right heart that is focused on the good of the patient to be successful at professional referral relationships
- You want to go into the community and develop relationships with other health practitioners by calling their offices, visiting their practices, and learning about what they do and how best you can help your patients by referring people to them (focus on 10 to start)
- Once you get to know them a bit invite them to a study group that you're going to do at your office one time per month on the same day and time
- After you have your first event identify 10 MORE practitioners to visit and invite to the study group for the next month
- Continue to do this every month for six months and by then you should have a strong collection of referral sources and a good group meeting in your practice every month
- Focus on discussing a topic that is of interest to a majority of the health professionals during the meeting.
- Clarify that this is NOT networking but instead is an opportunity to build relationships for the long term with other health professionals in the community
- Don't worry about exclusivity but instead invite multiple practitioners within the same discipline as different people will connect with others within the group regardless if there are multiple chiropractors, acupuncturists, physical therapists, dentists etc.
- You will need to refer many more patients to other health practitioners than you will receive back from them
- Once you develop a solid network of health professionals in your community you can get consistent new patient referrals from a variety of sources every month

BUILDING RELATIONSHIPS WITH OTHER
LOCAL BUSINESS OWNERS

Another way to develop consistent referrals is to build relationships with other local business owners. You can do this in networking events or business surveys but as Dr. Shawn Dill puts it:

"Networking is just creating relationships, sharing contacts, sharing information, sharing compassion, and developing that network of influence over the people that can influence your target market."

As we have discussed previously when you understand your ideal patient profile you can then look for people in your community such as coaches, support groups, gym owners or anyone else who might interact with your ideal patient on a regular basis.

Dr. Christina Meakim of San Francisco California is another doctor who has built some very significant relationships with other local business women and these relationships have developed into strong referral sources for her practice over many years. This is what she had to say about one of her favorite groups:

"My favorite one I joined was the Professional Women's Network. I found some of my best friends through that group and I met a lot of amazing people because entrepreneurs have a special kind of spirit."

If you can interact with other entrepreneurs, especially if they are similar to you or interact with a similar market that you are looking to attract, it could really be a great benefit to your practice.

CHAPTER FIFTEEN

DOMINATE ONLINE

How to Attract Your Ideal Patient Digitally

"A human being is drawn to clarity and simplicity and away from confusion."

– Donald Miller

In today's digital world it is crucial that your Upper Cervical Practice dominates online in your community. With the rise of Facebook, Pinterest, Instagram, YouTube, and other social networks and search engines like Google, Bing, and Yahoo your target market is online all the time and you can communicate with them wherever they are through their smartphones.

<u>Online marketing has been the number one way to generate new patients from external sources for 3 years in a row according to our Upper Cervical Practice surveys.</u>

The great thing about online marketing is that it has both short-term and long-term results and benefits. It is a cumulative approach, unlike spinal screenings, talks, health fairs or other one-off marketing approaches.

It also positions you as a respected expert who is providing a unique service to the community when done effectively.

When you have a comprehensive online marketing program in place focused on dominating online you can:

- Generate more new patients
- Increase referral conversion

- Build an email lead list for future marketing
- External event promotion
- Internal event promotion
- Improve patient education
- Increase retention
- Improve patient loyalty and compliance
- Increase reactivations
- Increase professional referrals
- Increase community awareness
- Improve online presence
- Increase collections

MINIMUM REQUIREMENTS NEEDED TO COMPETE ONLINE

At a minimum, here is what you need to compete online:

- Website
  - Mobile Responsive
  - Blogging Capabilities
- Facebook business page
  - (Not a profile only)
- YouTube channel for business
- Other social media
  - Pinterest
  - Instagram
- Claimed Google Listing
  - (So you can respond to reviews)
- Ways to attract and capture leads
- A system to follow up with leads
- A system to stay connected and top of mind with existing patients and gather testimonials and reviews

Upper Cervical Websites

When it comes to websites there are 3 keys that are important to communicate in five seconds or less:

1. Who You Are
2. What You Do
3. What to Do Next

1) *Who You Are*

Your website should represent you. I would recommend staying away from general chiropractic information and stock photos and videos that don't communicate who your unique team is to your ideal patient. But instead have images and videos with you, your team, and your patients that represent you and communicate to your ideal patient what you're all about.

2) *What You Do*

Your website should represent your unique practice. Not just a template of what a general chiropractic website company has created. But instead, have images and videos that communicate your unique Upper Cervical specific practice style. Why would you have a picture of someone doing a lower back adjustment when you do Upper Cervical work? This is just one example of the types of images we see on chiropractic websites all the time that don't communicate your unique Upper Cervical Practice style.

3) *What to Do Next*

Your website needs to be actionable. When someone lands on your website they need to be able to take action in five seconds or less to contact your office. The fact is that 80% of the people who land on your website will never scroll down so it is important to keep all the most important information above the fold on your website. It is essential that you have your phone number prominently displayed along with a call to action button that someone can click on to schedule a consultation.

Website Functionality

Along with communicating who you are, what you do, and what to do next, your website also needs to be functional for today's world. Approximately 60% of people who visit your website, will visit for the first time from a mobile device. So, it's absolutely vital that your website looks great on any mobile device including smartphones, tablets, etc.

If you are unsure about whether or not your website is currently mobile friendly put your website URL into this website from Google: https://www.google.com/webmasters/tools/mobile-friendly/.

It will tell you how mobile friendly your website is and ways to improve it. Along with your site being mobile friendly you also want to make sure that you can add additional content easily through a blog. Every website today should have blogging capabilities and have consistent content focused on your ideal patient being added to the website on a consistent basis.

We utilize WordPress to build all of our websites for clients as we believe that this is the most effective platform available today to build a website. WordPress websites are easy to blog on and are search engine friendly.

We think blogging is an important piece of the digital marketing picture and this is why it is included with all of our comprehensive marketing systems.

Optimizing Your Website for Conversion

You can have the most beautiful website in the world but if it doesn't convert visitors to leads and leads to new patients it adds' little to no value to your practice.

One of the most important aspects of having an optimized website is what we call the above the fold essentials. The fold is the portion of the website that you first see before you scroll down.

Having a phone number prominently displayed, a clear call to action on what to do next and an image that communicates who you are and what you do are crucial in this above the fold section.

We have found that staying away from stock images in this section is good. Utilizing images of the doctors working with patients has tested most effectively.

Logo and color scheme are also important factors when it comes to conversion on your website. And even the name of your practice can impact whether or not someone takes the next step to call or fill out a form to schedule a consultation.

We have already discussed these elements in more detail in chapter 8 when we discussed branding.

Optimizing Your Website for Search Engine Optimization

Once you have optimized your website for conversion the 2nd aspect of having an optimized website is optimizing it for search engines like Google, Bing, and Yahoo.

What is search engine optimization, or SEO?

Moz describes it as the process of increasing the number of visitors to a website by achieving a high rank in the search results of a search engine. The higher a website ranks in the results of a search, the greater the chance that users will visit the site. It is common practice for Internet users to not click past the first few pages of search results, therefore high rank in SERPs is essential for obtaining traffic for a site. SEO helps to ensure that a site is accessible to a search engine and improves the chances that the site will be indexed and favorably ranked by the search engine.

When it comes to search engine optimization for Upper Cervical Chiropractic websites it's crucial to have a very firm grasp on your keyword strategy.

There are many keywords that you might find yourself being ranked for that you may not want to have. Search engine optimization in many ways is about standing out from the crowd and connecting with the people who you want to attract into your practice.

So, the first step is to determine the keywords that your Upper Cervical Chiropractic practice website should rank for and the order of priority for those keywords. Then you can set up a strategy to rank your website for those keywords.

General chiropractor SEO strategy

Many online marketing companies will focus on ranking you for the keyword (Your town) chiropractor as a primary focus of their strategy.

A noted chiropractic Internet marketing consultant once said, "I imagine a person with one hand on their back and one hand on the mouse."

If this is the type of patient that you are primarily focused on seeing in your Upper Cervical Practice then without a doubt, you want to rank #1 for your town chiropractor and more including:

- (Your town) Chiropractor
- (Your town) (State Abbrev) Chiropractic
- (Your town) (State Abbrev.) Chiropractor
- (Your town) (State Abbrev.) Chiropractors
- (Your town) Chiropractic
- (Your town) Chiropractors
- Chiropractor (Your town)
- Chiropractors in (Your Town)
- Chiropractors (Your town)
- (Your zip code) Chiropractor
- (Your zip code) Chiropractic

- Chiropractor (Your zip code)
- (Your zip code) Chiropractic
- Chiropractic (Your zip code)
- Chiropractic Office (Your zip code)
- Chiropractic Office (Your town)
- Chiropractic (Your town)
- Chiropractic Doctor (Your town)
- Chiropractor Doctor (Your town)
- Chiropractic Physician (Your town)

People who search for these types of keywords are typically focused on relief only and likely already have a predefined notion of what type of care they need (i.e. "I just need someone to crack my back").

So you may think twice about primarily focusing on this general Chiropractor SEO strategy.

Prioritizing your keyword strategy
Now I'm not suggesting that there is no value associated with the general chiropractic search engine optimization strategy outlined above but I am suggesting that for an Upper Cervical Chiropractic Practice this should not be your primary search engine optimization strategy.

Upper Cervical Chiropractors typically want to attract high-quality new patients that will stay, pay and refer. If you want to attract these types of new patients, then a good SEO prioritization is the following:

1. Upper Cervical/Technique Specific Keywords For Your Local Area
2. Condition Specific Keywords for Your Local Area
3. General Chiropractic Keywords for Your Local Area

The best way we have found to search engine optimize an Upper Cervical Chiropractic website is to focus first on Upper Cervical and technique related keywords such as:

- Upper Cervical Chiropractor (Your town)
- Upper Cervical Chiropractors in (Your Town)
- Upper Cervical Chiropractors (Your town)
- (Your town) Upper Cervical Chiropractor
- (Your town) (State Abbrev) Upper Cervical Chiropractic

- (Your town) (State Abbrev.) Upper Cervical Chiropractor
- (Your town) (State Abbrev.) Upper Cervical Chiropractors
- (Your town) Upper Cervical Chiropractic
- (Your town) Upper Cervical Chiropractors
- Upper Cervical Care (Your town)
- Upper Cervical (Your town)
- (your technique) Chiropractic (Your town)
- (your technique) Chiropractor (Your town)

For these keywords, every Upper Cervical Practice in a smaller market should be ranking #1 on page #1 in Google search results. In a medium or large competitive market, you would want to at least be ranked in the top 3 for your area.

Ranking for these keywords will make sure that anyone in your local area who is looking for an Upper Cervical Specialist or more specifically a specialist in your Upper Cervical technique such as NUCCA, Atlas Orthogonal, Orthospinology, Blair, etc. will find you.

Condition Specific SEO for Chiropractors
Once your website has been search engine optimized for the Upper Cervical related keywords above, the next focus should be on condition-specific keywords that will connect you with your ideal patient.

These are the keywords that someone with a particular condition would be searching for in your area. Now you have to be careful with your local regulatory agency when it comes to the use of certain words on your website that patients would be searching for such as specialist, treatment, cure etc.

If your ideal patient is a migraine sufferer then you would want to make sure that you are ranking for migraine-related keywords such as:

- migraine relief (your town)
- migraine relief (Your Town) (State Abbrev)
- (Your town) (State Abbrev) migraine relief
- (your town) migraine relief

This would apply to any condition that you would like to help more patients with like vertigo, fibromyalgia, TMJ, post-concussion syndrome, etc.

You want to make sure that you are regularly writing blog content and featuring pages on your website that are specific to these keywords for the different conditions or types of patients on which you would like to focus.

Cornerstone content

It is essential to keep writing blog content that is focused on your target conditions. The next step is to establish some specific blog posts as cornerstone content.

Cornerstone content should include:

- A minimum of 900 words
- A detailed explanation of the condition
- Information about the Upper Cervical approach and why it helps so many people who suffer from this condition.

Once you have a good cornerstone article written for your target keyword, next you want to create other blog articles with related keywords and create backlinks to your cornerstone article.

You should also link all of your cornerstone content articles to your homepage, this will show Google that these are the most important articles on your website.

Having a well-thought-out and effective search engine optimization strategy in place for your Upper Cervical Practice will help you attract high-quality new patients for years to come.

Upper Cervical Directories

Another aspect of search engine optimization that is important is to make sure that you have plenty of backlinks. Backlinks are when you have a link from another website to your website. One way to increase your backlinks while also getting more exposure from potential new patients is to add your practice to as many directories as possible.

There are 3 main types of Upper Cervical Directories available including:

1. Technique Directories
2. Advocate Directories
3. General Upper Cervical Directories

Technique directories

Directories for individual techniques would include NUCCA, Atlas Orthogonal, Knee Chest, Blair, Orthospinology, Advanced Orthogonal, QSM3 etc. If you practice one of these techniques I highly recommend that you become a member if you are not already and that you are listed in their directory.

For example, NUCCA is the most searched for Upper Cervical related keyword on Google. If you practice NUCCA make sure that you are keeping your membership in good standing not only for the fact that it will help you to be a better doctor but also so you can be listed in their directory and receive patients who are specifically looking for a NUCCA Doctor in your area.

This would also apply to other techniques as well. Here is a list of some of the main Upper Cervical technique directories for your convenience:

- http://www.nucca.org/
- http://www.atlasorthogonality.com/
- http://www.kcucs.com/
- http://www.blairchiropractic.com/
- http://orthospinology.org/
- http://www.advancedorthogonal.com/
- http://www.qsm3.com/

Advocate directory

The next directory to focus on is one created by Upper Cervical advocate Greg Buchanan. This website is fantastic for third-party endorsement of what you do. Make sure that you are listed on this important directory. http://www.upcspine.com/prac1.asp

General upper cervical directories

And lastly, you want to be listed on general Upper Cervical directories such as uppercervicalcare.com and upper-cervical.com. Uppercervicalcare.com is especially important as it shows up on the first page of Google for a variety of Upper Cervical related keywords.

Dr. Ian Bulow also has a very comprehensive directory of Upper Cervical Doctors on his website. I believe you have to be in good standing with your technique certification in order to appear in his directory.

Here are the links to the general upper cervical directories we recommend:

- http://uppercervicalcare.com/
- http://www.upper-cervical.com/html/directory.html#VT
- http://uppercervicalawareness.com/find-a-doctor/
- http://revivepittsburgh.com/referral-list/

How to list your practice

It is important that you list your practice on these directories the same way that Google has you listed (you also want to make sure that your website lists you the same way).

Make sure you include:

- Name (Dr. John Smith)
- Practice Name (Smith Spinal Care)
- Address
- Phone Number
- Website

Going through the process of getting listed on as many of these directories as possible will provide you with backlinks and other search engine optimization benefits but most importantly qualified patients who are looking specifically for Upper Cervical care.

If you are really not interested in spending the time and energy necessary to optimize your website for conversion and search then we would highly recommend purchasing an Upper Cervical Specific Website from us. Our websites are completely optimized for conversion and search engines, are mobile ready and will save you valuable time.

You can learn more about our upper cervical websites at www.uppercervicalmarketing.com.

Once you have optimized your website for conversion and search engines you will see much more return on your investment when it comes to your website.

However, if you do not have a comprehensive online marketing program in place that utilizes key strategies specific to your practice, you will get limited results with your online marketing efforts regardless of how great your website may be.

Case Studies

The benefits of dominating online in your area are tremendous. Whether you are in the US in a small town, a medium-sized market, a large competitive market, or an international market such as Canada, Australia, New Zealand or the Philippines, online marketing can absolutely change your practice.

Below I'm going to highlight some of the stories of clients that we have worked with who were in different types of markets and have all seen tremendous success. You can find even more stories like this on our website.

Dr. Christopher Perkins – Detroit, Michigan (large competitive market)

Dr. Perkins was tired of spending his nights and weekends doing screenings, dinner talks, lunch and learns and other "feet on the street" types of marketing. Since he had two small children it was important to him to find a way that he could generate new patients without these types of time intensive marketing approaches. It was also important for him to have a consistent source of new patients so that he could have less variability in his income. Online marketing has proved to be the answer to both of his desires.

Dr. Perkins has been able to generate 10 to 15 new patients per month from the Internet and has had record collections month after month without screenings or other one-off marketing approaches. New patients consistently call his office from his strong Google, Facebook, YouTube, Pinterest, and Instagram presences. The patients he receives from the Internet have been great patients who are willing to pay cash for his services and are pre-educated about Upper Cervical care. He has a consistently high closing rate with these patients of about 90%. These new patients have also become a great referral source for him to improve his practice even more.

Dr. Joe Breuwet – Honolulu, Hawaii (medium-sized market)

Dr. Breuwet was also tired of the new patients he was getting from screenings and wanted a better option to generate new patients who were of a higher quality.

Dr. Joe now sees 8 to 15 new patients per month from the Internet. He has also noticed that the patients he gets from our Upper Cervical Marketing System are much higher quality than any other patients he has ever had from any type of marketing. He is converting at close to 90% on these new patients.

Dr. Kurt Sherwood – Renton, Washington (medium-sized market)

Dr. Sherwood has consistently seen high-quality new patients from the Internet for over four years utilizing our system. He just set a record for new patients for the first quarter of this year because of his strong Internet presence!

Dr. Brett Gottlieb – Fair Oaks, California (small market)

Dr. Gottlieb has been consistently attracting high-quality new patients from the Internet for over three years with our system. He is now seen as a migraine and vertigo expert in his area because of his consistent Internet marketing. Professional and patient referrals have increased and consistently sees 15 to 20 new patients per month from the Internet alone.

Dr. Casey Weerheim – Sioux Falls, South Dakota (small market)

Dr. Weerheim is NOW able to focus on patient care instead of marketing. Dr. Casey was going out looking for patients at screenings and talks but now they call him. He sees 8 to 15 new patients from online marketing every month.

Dr. Kristen McClure – Charlevoix, Michigan (small market)

Dr. McClure has been able to triple her new patients and her practice through Internet marketing!

Dr. Geoff Besso – Stow, Ohio (small market)

Dr. Besso has been able to change his culture by consistently attracting patients with chronic health conditions who have not been able to find help anywhere else.

He consistently sees approximately 10 new patients per month from his small community and generates a ton of referrals from these patients as well.

Dr. Miguel Flores – Manila, Philippines (large international market)

Dr. Flores and his brother Dr. Gabriel Flores have seen incredible results with our Upper Cervical Marketing System. He has consistently set collections records, has a 2 to 3-week waiting list in his original clinic in Manila and has consistently seen between 40 to 80 new patients per month from the Internet. He was also able to open a second clinic in Alabang, Philippines and is consistently seeing over 40 new patients per month from the Internet from his second program as well. Dr. Flores has also been featured on CNN Philippines as a migraine expert as a result of his online marketing program.

Dr. Benjamin Kuhn – Edmonton, Alberta Canada (large international market)

Dr. Kuhn has been seeing 10 to 20 new patients per month with a 20 to 1 return on investment from our Upper Cervical Marketing System!

Doing online marketing yourself?

If you are currently attempting to do online marketing yourself for your Upper Cervical Practice or are having one of your team members do it I want to encourage you to delegate your online marketing.

Of course, I am biased. I believe strongly in our services, and not just because of all the doctors who I've mentioned above who have had tremendous results.

But also because I was once in practice and I know that I did not have the time, energy or know how to do online marketing effectively for my own Upper Cervical Practice at the time.

Online marketing is very complicated and is constantly changing. To keep up with it is very time-consuming.

But for the cost of a part-time team member, you can partner with Upper Cervical Marketing.

Our Upper Cervical Marketing System is focused on producing the following features and benefits:

- Attract qualified leads with chronic health conditions
- Turn leads from the internet into new patients
- Delight your existing patients to promote retention, reactivations,

testimonials, reviews, and referral conversion.

- Create high-quality Upper Cervical Specific content for you including:

  o Facebook ads, videos, e-books, landing pages, blogs and email autoresponders
  o Whiteboard video marketing
  o Search Engine Optimization (SEO)
  o Online review generation

- Personal attention and ongoing support/insights from our Upper Cervical Marketing Team

To see if our system is a fit for your practice simply give us a call at 877-252-1230 and select option one and we can do a quick Upper Cervical Practice Health Screening. In five minutes we can see whether or not it makes sense to take a deeper dive into your practice with the possibility of partnering together.

CHAPTER SIXTEEN

KEEP UP WITH GROWTH

There Is No Status Quo

"Change is inevitable. Growth is optional."

— John Maxwell

This last chapter is going to focus on growth. Growth in an Upper Cervical Practice can either be a blessing or a curse.

If your practice is not ready to grow and it grows quickly it can actually negatively impact your practice and cause you to lose a tremendous amount of ground.

Do you ever feel like you're barely keeping your head above water?

This can be the reality of growth.

You may feel like you can never keep up and are constantly running around trying to do everything.

But it doesn't have to be this way.

When you are strategic about the growth of your Upper Cervical Practice you can prepare for and easily respond to growth.

Let's look at five keys to thrive in the midst of a growing practice.

#1 CONFRONT THE BRUTAL FACTS
WITHOUT LOSING FAITH

Earlier in the book, we discussed the importance of embracing the Stockdale Paradox for your personal growth. It is also important to embrace the same paradox for your practice growth.

To keep up with growth you must be both a realist and an optimist at the same time.

Confront the brutal facts of what has led to your current reality while having the faith to believe that things will be better in the future.

It's important to remember to consistently and thoroughly evaluate all aspects of your business to see where you can be more efficient or effective.

#2 PREPARE THE LAND FOR RAIN

In the movie *Facing the Giants* one of the characters Mr. Bridges shares a story with the coach:

"I heard of a story of two farmers praying to God for the rain to come. Both prayed but only one prepared the land. Who do you think trusted God more to send the rain?"

Earlier in this book, we discussed the importance of setting goals. Once you have set your goals you need to put systems in place **now** to help you reach your goal in the **future**.

For instance, if your goal is for your practice to see 150 patient visits per week then it's important that you determine what your practice will look like when you are seeing 150 patient visits per week including:

Growth Rate
How quickly do you expect to grow to that point?

If you are at 100 patient visits per week do you expect to be at 150 in 3 months? 1 year? 2 years?

This will determine the timing of everything else.

Team Members
How many team members will you need in order to see 150 patient visits per week? Do you need an additional CA? An associate? An office manager?

Equipment
Will you need additional tables? Will you need to upgrade to digital x-ray?

Office Space
Will you need to move? Will you need more space? Will you need to redesign space that you have?

Leadership/Management Qualities
What type of leader do you need to be in order to manage an office of that size? Do you need additional coaching or consulting?

Outsourcing
Are you currently leaving your office to do all of your marketing through screenings, talks etc.? Would it be more beneficial for you to outsource your marketing which would free you up to be in the office taking care patients?

Have You Created An Org Chart?
One of the most effective ways to visualize what your practice will look like for any particular goal is to create an organizational chart for what your practice will look like at that time.

Here are some things to keep in mind about org charts:

- NOT just for large corporations
- What does your practice look like when it's done?
- How many boxes are you in and how can you get out of some of those boxes?
- Which boxes are most important to move out of first?

#3 HIRE AHEAD TO AVOID FEELING OVERWHELMED

Strategically hiring at the right times is also key to keeping up with growth.

Most of the time we are reacting to growth rather than preparing for and receiving it.

To keep up with the growth you want to hire ahead instead of hiring behind.

Most of the time doctors are hiring people 3 to 6 months later than they should.

Hire the right people based on attitude, cultural fit, and core values and avoid the wrong people when hiring CA'S, Office Managers, and Associates.

#4 USE TECHNOLOGY TO GROW SMART

If you have a good practice that is building...the right technology accelerator can help you break through to the next level.

Digital X-Ray is one of the most effective technology accelerators for the Upper Cervical Practice. Your ability to process new patients and x-ray retakes in an Upper Cervical Practice are keys to efficiency and digital x-ray can help tremendously.

Chirotouch or other similar patient management software can help streamline your office operations and move away from paper.

#5 DELEGATE AND ELEVATE

As we discussed in a previous chapter a key to growing is learning how to delegate and elevate your team. You especially want to focus on delegating those tasks and responsibilities that you don't love and/or you are not great at.

Many times you may be stepping over dollars to pick up pennies in your practice by not delegating.

Dr. Kyrie Kleinfelter of St. Charles Illinois has a developed fantastic practice through delegation and elevation. Over the years, Dr. Kleinfelter has established solid systems, a great associate program, and a wonderful team. This flexibility has allowed Dr. Kleinfelter to enjoy five maternity leaves and long vacations with her family because of the solid systems and delegation practices she has had in her practice. On episode 36 of the podcast we discussed how she has been able to balance 3 extremely important goals:

- Taking really good care of people (high touch)
- Delivering high-quality care (high-quality)
- Helping a lot of people (high-volume)

At one point in the conversation, I asked her if there was a resistance between those three goals and this is what she said:

Dr. Kleinfelter: "I don't know that there is a resistance between the goals. I think my vision was so strong and clear that it meshed together before I even started it but there's a lot of hard work that goes behind it. There are always challenges. But if you have the strong guiding vision, you're heading in that direction...not that the road isn't bumpy."

She went on to emphasize the importance of maintaining a personal connection with patients while delivering high-quality care in a high-volume practice is extremely dependent on having strong systems in place and a solid team. Her thoughts are congruent with what we have talked about throughout this book and each of these goals is so important when it comes to keeping up with growth.

TAKING YOUR PRACTICE FROM GOOD TO GREAT

Many Upper Cervical Practices are good.

But to be truly great like Dr. Kleinfelter's practice **an Upper Cervical Practice must move from a job to a business.**

A business can go on without you and can even thrive when you are not there.

For instance, Dr. Kleinfelter's practice is so solid that she can take a month off during the year to spend time vacationing with her husband and five kids and her practice does not miss a beat.

That is a truly great practice!

In Jim Collins terrific book *Good to Great*, he discusses the key elements of companies that have been able to move from good companies to enduring great companies.

Step 1:
Become a Great Leader

Your ability to lead others will determine whether or not your practice becomes truly great.

Jim Collins found that the leaders of great companies were Level 5 Leaders.

The first 4 levels are:

Level 1 = A Highly Capable Individual

Level 2 = A Contributing Team Member

Level 3 = A Competent Manager

Level 4 = An Effective Leader

Most Upper Cervical Doctors are highly capable individuals who have become contributing team members. If you have a good practice than you are likely a competent manager and may be an effective leader. But to take your practice from good to great you must become a level 5 leader.

A Level 5 Leader builds enduring greatness of his or her practice through a paradoxical blend of personal humility and professional will.

There are several characteristics of a Level 5 Leader that you need to embrace and strive towards on a daily basis if you want your practice to go from good to great.

- **#1 Humility**. There's a big difference between confidence and arrogance. Humility is a key to building a great practice. It means being humble about who you are, about where you are in the world, and about the things that you need to learn.

- **#2 Honesty**. You need to be honest with yourself and others. Be honest about the problems and the issues that you're facing in your life and in your practice. It's so easy to lie to ourselves and sometimes it's easier to believe the lie than it is to be truly honest with ourselves.

- **#3 Results-oriented**. Being results oriented is key for level 5 leaders. Focus on attaining results through humility and honesty.

- **#4 Workmanlike Diligence.** Level 5 leaders are more plow horse then show horse. Diligence is having excellence in the ordinary over time to produce steady and consistent results.

A great analogy that Jim Collins mentions in *Good to Great* is the mirror and window analogy, and it's a great picture of who a level 5 leader is, and who you should aspire to be if you want to take your practice from good to great.

The mirror and window analogy goes like this:

When things are going well, level 5 leaders look outside the window and contribute some success to other outside factors: the organization, their team members, good fortune, etc.

So, when things are going well, you look outside, you look for the reasons why that's happening outside of yourself. That's the humble level 5 leader.

The second part of the analogy is the mirror part when things do not go well, level 5 leaders look in the mirror. They take responsibility. They do not make excuses or blame others.

This is a key to being both a realistic and humble leader at the same time.

Step 2:
First Who Then What

For Upper Cervical Doctors it is crucial to hire the right CA's and Associates for your team as we have discussed in detail in previous chapters. Without the right people on your team, you will not become a great company.

Step 3:
Focus on Your Hedgehog Concept

What is the Hedgehog Concept? It's based on the famous essay by Isaiah Berlin, "The Hedgehog and the Fox" which describes how the world is divided into two types. The fox knows many things. The fox is a very cunning creature, able to devise a myriad of complex strategies to sneak attack upon the hedgehog.

The hedgehog on the other hand, knows one big thing, rolling up into a perfect little ball thus becoming a sphere of sharp spikes, pointing outward in all directions. The hedgehog always wins despite the different tactics the fox uses. This is an illustration of the power of focus.

For your Upper Cervical Practice, the *Good to Great* Hedgehog Concept is the intersection of three overlapping circles:

1. **What are you deeply passionate about?**

   (Your ideal patient)

2. **What can your practice be the best in the world at?**

   (Serving your ideal patient with your upper cervical niche)

3. **What drives your economic engine?**

   (Office Visit Average OVA)

The answers to these 3 questions will help you to determine a focus for your practice that will allow you to move from good to great.

Step 4:
Develop a Culture of Discipline

When you and your team are disciplined to focus on becoming masters of Upper Cervical Practice and not a "jack of all trades" practice, you will be able to take your practice from good to great.

CONCLUSION

Hopefully, in this book, you have learned from the world's top Upper Cervical Doctors what it takes to be successful.

Now, you must take action.

As Sir Walter Scott said so well:

> *"I can give you a six-word formula for success:*
> *think things through – then follow through"*

Throughout this book, I have given you a lot to think about when it comes to your personal, practice, and growth mastery now it's time to follow through.

Information without implementation leads to frustration.

Begin to implement slowly. Make a list of 12 things you want to implement from this book and then set out to implement one per month over the next 12 months.

Doing that alone will have a dramatic impact on your practice!

Next make another list of 12 more things to implement and implement that over the next 12 months and so forth.

To help you with the implementation of the principles and practices in this book we have developed a companion study course called **UCP Master Academy**. This study group contains in-depth webinars about each chapter with tools and resources to help you execute strategies, email Q&A availability, and exclusive access to a private Facebook group for accountability and community with other doctors and students on the journey to become Upper Cervical Practice Masters.

To learn more about the **UCP Master Academy** go to http://uppercervicalpracticemastery.com/academy.

There is a ton of great information in this book that you can use to become an Upper Cervical Practice Master and to grow a great practice for the sake of your patients, your community, your team, your family, and you personally.

Be sure you subscribe to The Upper Cervical Marketing Podcast on iTunes, Stitcher or wherever you like to listen to podcasts. You can also listen online at www.uppercervicalmarketing.com/podcast. On the website, you will also find loads of free resources including many of the resources discussed in this book, on-demand webinars, hundreds of blog posts, and so much more. Our goal at Upper Cervical Marketing is to help you free up your time, increase your collections, and love your marketing!

I sincerely hope you will take the challenge to become one of the world's top Upper Cervical Doctors because we need to work together to take Upper Cervical to the world!

References and Resources

Introduction
http://www.uppercervicalmarketing.com/podcast

http://uppercervicalmarketing.com/blog/2016surveyresults/

http://uppercervicalmarketing.com/blog/2017-upper-cervical-practice-survey-results/

CHAPTER 1 Evaluate Your Life
https://assessments.michaelhyatt.com/lifescore/

http://uppercervicalmarketing.com/blog/ucm-048-how-dr-christine-zapata-built-dream-clinic/

CHAPTER 2 Build a Mindset That Wins
http://uppercervicalmarketing.com/blog/ucm-047-how-dr-steve-judson-purpose-driven-highly-successful-practice/

http://uppercervicalmarketing.com/blog/dr-julie-mayer-hunt-and-having-purpose-in-chiropractic-marketing/

http://uppercervicalmarketing.com/blog/ucm-044-power-intentionality-revolutionized-dr-ed-gigliottis-practice/

http://uppercervicalmarketing.com/blog/dr-justin-brown-confidence-certainty-and-500-patient-visits-per-week/

http://uppercervicalmarketing.com/blog/ucm-015-dr-justin-brown-champion-mindset-practice-life/

http://uppercervicalmarketing.com/blog/analysis-paralysis-killing-your-upper-cervical-practice-growth/

http://uppercervicalmarketing.com/blog/not-allowing-upper-cervical-practice-grow/

http://uppercervicalmarketing.com/blog/episode6/

Good to Great by Jim Collins

https://ndoherty.com/stockdale-paradox/

http://uppercervicalmarketing.com/blog/ucm-037-dr-kurt-sherwood-combined-vision-perseverance-strategic-marketing-grow-successful-upper-cervical-practice/

http://uppercervicalmarketing.com/blog/3-ways-arrogance-success-can-stall-upper-cervical-practice-growth/

http://uppercervicalmarketing.com/blog/dr-terry-mccoskey-keeping-fun-in-your-chiropractic-marketing/

http://uppercervicalmarketing.com/blog/dr-drew-hall-and-keeping-the-passion-in-your-upper-cervical-practice/

http://uppercervicalmarketing.com/blog/dr-christina-meakim-and-how-to-grow-an-upper-cervical-practice-with-personal-touch/

CHAPTER 3 Cultivate Your Habits

http://uppercervicalmarketing.com/blog/10-keys-to-grow-your-practice-in-2016-that-require-zero-talent-but-most-people-wont-do/

CHAPTER 4 Cast Your Practice Vision

http://uppercervicalmarketing.com/blog/developing-your-core-values-vision-and-mission-for-your-upper-cervical-practice/

https://hbr.org/2002/07/make-your-values-mean-something

http://deliveringhappiness.com/

http://uppercervicalmarketing.com/blog/dr-terry-mccoskey-keeping-fun-in-your-chiropractic-marketing/

http://uppercervicalmarketing.com/blog/ucm-016-dr-ian-davis-tremayne-creating-upper-cervical-revolution-building-practice-dreams/

http://uppercervicalmarketing.com/blog/ucm-042-build-dream-practice-focusing-executing-vision-dr-christopher-wolff/

Built to Last by Jim Collins and Jerry Porras

http://uppercervicalmarketing.com/blog/how-to-create-incredible-practice-results-by-focusing-on-your-bhag/

https://www.americanexpress.com/us/small-business/openforum/articles/how-to-set-a-bhag-1/

https://www.linkedin.com/pulse/best-practices-achieve-your-bhag-stephen-lynch/

https://www.mindtools.com/pages/article/smart-goals.htm

http://uppercervicalmarketing.com/blog/dr-larry-arbeitman-and-how-to-build-a-team-to-grow-your-upper-cervical-practice/

http://uppercervicalmarketing.com/blog/episode1/

CHAPTER 5 Master Your Upper Cervical Technique
http://www.icauppercervical.com/Diplomate-Program

http://uppercervicalmarketing.com/blog/7-practice-success-keys-i-have-learned-from-top-upper-cervical-doctors/

E Myth Revisited by Michael Gerber

CHAPTER 6 Succeed with Your Team
The Ideal Team Player by Patrick Lencioni

Good to Great by Jim Collins

https://discprofile.com/what-is-disc/overview/

https://www.daveramsey.com/store/budgeting-tools/online-tools/disc-assessment-test/proddisc.html

http://uppercervicalmarketing.com/blog/ucm-026-invest-team-promote-excellence-practice-dr-jamie-cramer/

http://uppercervicalmarketing.com/blog/ucm-018-succeed-associate-relationships-upper-cervical-practice-dr-noel-lloyd/

http://uppercervicalmarketing.com/blog/dr-nick-tedder-and-the-importance-of-mentorship-for-your-upper-cervical-practice/

http://uppercervicalmarketing.com/blog/dr-noel-lloyd-and-win-win-associate-programs-new-patients-and-more/

CHAPTER 7 Run Your Upper Cervical Business
Traction by Gino Wickman

http://uppercervicalmarketing.com/blog/ucm-020-develop-systems-improve-efficiency-effectiveness-upper-cervical-practice-dr-michael-lenarz/

http://uppercervicalmarketing.com/blog/what-would-happen-to-your-upper-cervical-practice-if-you-were-injured/

http://uppercervicalmarketing.com/blog/ucm-014-marty-paradise-certified-e-myth-business-coach-entrepreneurial-myth-upper-cervical-doctors-struggling-practices/

http://adjustingattitudes.com/technique-addresses-1-problem-chiropractic-retention-are-you-using-it

Profit First by Mike Michalowicz

CHAPTER 8 Set the Stage for Success

http://www.dynamicchiropractic.com/digital/index.php?i=1229&Page=40

http://uppercervicalmarketing.com/blog/defining-your-ideal-patient-for-your-upper-cervical-practice/

https://www.business2community.com/marketing/wtf-happened-target-markets-buyer-persona

https://blog.hubspot.com/marketing/buyer-persona-questions

http://uppercervicalmarketing.com/blog/name-upper-cervical-practice-can-impact-marketing/

http://chiropractic.prosepoint.net/88653

http://www.dynamicchiropractic.com/mpacms/dc/article.php?id=52038

http://news.gallup.com/poll/184910/majority-say-chiropractic-works-neck-back-pain.aspx

http://uppercervicalmarketing.com/blog/logo-color-scheme-can-impact-upper-cervical-marketing/

http://uppercervicalmarketing.com/blog/creating-culture-social-proof-upper-cervical-practice/

http://www.tandfonline.com/doi/abs/10.1080/01449290500330448

https://www.entrepreneur.com/slideshow/299455

https://www.entrepreneur.com/article/21774

http://www.emeraldinsight.com/doi/abs/10.1108/00251740610673332

https://www.optimus01.co.za/psychology-of-colours/

http://uppercervicalmarketing.com/blog/why-would-an-upper-cervical-doctor-use-general-chiropractic-brochures/

http://uppercervicalmarketing.com/blog/how-to-use-the-7-learning-styles-to-communicate-effectively-in-your-upper-cervical-practice/

CHAPTER 9 Become a Master Communicator

http://uppercervicalmarketing.com/blog/how-to-use-the-7-learning-styles-to-communicate-effectively-in-your-upper-cervical-practice/

http://uppercervicalmarketing.com/blog/episode3/

http://uppercervicalmarketing.com/blog/episode1/

http://uppercervicalmarketing.com/blog/dr-kerry-johnson-and-using-tools-to-grow-your-upper-cervical-practice/

http://uppercervicalmarketing.com/blog/ucm-033-communicating-upper-cervical-passion-help-people-dr-dennis-young/

http://uppercervicalmarketing.com/blog/dr-todd-osborne-and-communicating-the-upper-cervical-message/

http://uppercervicalmarketing.com/blog/ucm-017-dr-todd-osborne-avoid-common-mistakes-doctors-make-consult-exam-report/

http://uppercervicalmarketing.com/blog/dr-robert-brooks-and-communication-in-upper-cervical-marketing/

http://uppercervicalmarketing.com/blog/ucm-034-avoid-3-common-mistakes-doctors-make-workshops-individual-communication-keith-wassung/

http://uppercervicalmarketing.com/blog/episode5/

http://www.dyslexiavictoriaonline.com/learning-style-auditory-visual-kinesthetic-dyslexics/

https://www.learning-styles-online.com/style/visual-spatial/

https://www.learning-styles-online.com/style/aural-auditory-musical/

https://www.learning-styles-online.com/style/verbal-linguistic/

https://www.learning-styles-online.com/style/physical-bodily-kinesthetic/

https://www.learning-styles-online.com/style/logical-mathematical/

https://www.learning-styles-online.com/style/social-interpersonal/

https://www.learning-styles-online.com/style/solitary-intrapersonal/

https://mymisalignment.com/

https://www.learning-styles-online.com/inventory/questions.php

http://uppercervicalmarketing.com/shop/

https://www.classy.org/blog/tips-for-appealing-to-every-type-of-communicator/

http://uppercervicalmarketing.com/product-category/chartsposters/

CHAPTER 10 Keep Patients on Track
http://uppercervicalmarketing.com/blog/the-forgotten-part-of-marketing-for-your-upper-cervical-practice/

CHAPTER 11 Plan Your Marketing for Growth
http://uppercervicalmarketing.com/blog/ucm-024-overcoming-sales-marketing-taboos-grow-practice-2017/

http://uppercervicalmarketing.com/blog/dr-michael-lenarz-and-the-chiropractic-marketing-life-cycle/

http://www.businessinsider.com/corporations-ad-spending-2011-6?op=1

http://uppercervicalmarketing.com/blog/how-much-should-your-chiropractic-marketing-budget-be/

http://uppercervicalmarketing.com/blog/how-to-budget-for-your-chiropractic-marketing-based-on-market/

http://uppercervicalmarketing.com/budgetcalculator/

http://uppercervicalmarketing.com/blog/3-essentials-success-chiropractic-marketing-program/

http://uppercervicalmarketing.com/blog/how-to-design-your-2018-chiropractic-marketing-plan-for-growth/

http://uppercervicalmarketing.com/blog/ucm-043-dr-chris-slininger-used-strategic-planning-build-multimillion-dollar-practice/

http://uppercervicalmarketing.com/blog/ucm-023-planning-best-year-practice-2017/

http://uppercervicalmarketing.com/blog/top-10-chiropractic-marketing-ideas-2017/

http://uppercervicalmarketing.com/blog/best-ways-to-promote-your-chiropractic-practice/

http://uppercervicalmarketing.com/blog/the-dos-and-donts-of-marketing-for-chiropractors/

http://uppercervicalmarketing.com/blog/7-ways-to-integrate-your-chiropractic-marketing-to-grow-your-practice-in-2018/

http://uppercervicalmarketing.com/blog/how-to-do-an-integrated-fb-live-new-patient-orientation-class-to-generate-more-referrals/

CHAPTER 12 Own the 3R's of Internal Practice Success

http://uppercervicalmarketing.com/blog/ucm-028-use-referral-statements-every-patient-every-visit-generate-ongoing-referrals-dr-jon-baker/

http://uppercervicalmarketing.com/blog/ucm-025-dr-terry-mccoskey-building-cash-practice-referrals-re-activations/

http://uppercervicalmarketing.com/blog/how-to-increase-referrals-to-your-upper-cervical-practice/

http://adjustingattitudes.com/technique-addresses-1-problem-chiropractic-retention-are-you-using-it

http://uppercervicalmarketing.com/blog/the-forgotten-part-of-marketing-for-your-upper-cervical-practice/

http://uppercervicalmarketing.com/blog/the-3-essentials-of-internal-marketing-for-chiropractors/

http://uppercervicalmarketing.com/blog/improve-re-activations-referrals-upper-cervical-practice/

http://uppercervicalmarketing.com/blog/ucm-025-dr-terry-mccoskey-building-cash-practice-referrals-re-activations/

CHAPTER 13 Build a Positive Practice Reputation
Influence by Robert Cialdini

http://uppercervicalmarketing.com/blog/creating-culture-social-proof-upper-cervical-practice/

http://uppercervicalmarketing.com/blog/still-less-25-google-reviews-need/

http://uppercervicalmarketing.com/blog/creative-way-to-get-more-reviews-for-your-upper-cervical-practice/

http://uppercervicalmarketing.com/blog/how-to-get-a-good-video-testimonial-for-your-upper-cervical-practice/

http://uppercervicalmarketing.com/blog/how-to-get-a-good-video-testimonial-for-your-upper-cervical-practice-part-2/

http://uppercervicalmarketing.com/blog/why-yelp-reviews-get-filtered-for-your-upper-cervical-practice/

https://www.brightlocal.com/learn/local-consumer-review-survey/#Q12

CHAPTER 14 Grow Your Practice Through Professional Referrals
http://uppercervicalmarketing.com/blog/dr-jeff-scholten-and-being-professional-in-chiropractic-marketing-part-1-of-2/

http://uppercervicalmarketing.com/blog/ucm-040-dr-giancarlo-licata-built-integrative-community-health-professionals-can/

http://uppercervicalmarketing.com/blog/dr-shawn-dill-and-building-relationships-to-grow-your-upper-cervical-practice/

http://uppercervicalmarketing.com/blog/dr-christina-meakim-and-how-to-grow-an-upper-cervical-practice-with-personal-touch/

CHAPTER 15 Dominate Online

https://uppercervicalmarketing.com/blog/seo-for-chiropractors-attract-high-quality-new-patients/

https://uppercervicalmarketing.com/blog/optimize-upper-cervical-website-conversion-search/

https://uppercervicalmarketing.com/blog/basics-of-search-engine-optimization-for-your-upper-cervical-website/

https://www.revenuelabs.com/blog/chiropractic-case-study

https://uppercervicalmarketing.com/blog/are-you-listed-in-these-important-upper-cervical-directories/

https://uppercervicalmarketing.com/upper-cervical-chiropractic-websites/

http://uppercervicalmarketing.com/blog/10-chiropractic-internet-marketing-experts-share-whats-working-in-2016-and-beyond/

http://uppercervicalmarketing.com/blog/7-chiropractic-internet-marketing-experts-share-whats-working-2017-beyond/

http://uppercervicalmarketing.com/upper-cervical-chiropractic-marketing-case-studies/

CHAPTER 16 Keep Up With Growth

5 Ways to Keep up with Growth in Your Upper Cervical Practice
https://app.webinarjam.net/register/33369/286c43609f

http://uppercervicalmarketing.com/blog/ucm-036-grow-high-quality-high-volume-high-touch-practice-dr-kyrie-kleinfelter/

Good to Great by Jim Collins

Taking Your Practice from Good to Great

http://uppercervicalmarketing.com/blog/episode4/

ABOUT THE AUTHOR

Dr. Bill Davis lives just north of San Diego California with his wife and three children. Dr. Davis graduated from Los Angeles College of Chiropractic in 2005 and was a highly successful Upper Cervical Chiropractor until a mountain biking accident in November 2011 resulted in a spinal cord injury that left him paralyzed and unable to practice. Since 2013, Dr. Davis and his team at Upper Cervical Marketing have helped over 200 Upper Cervical Doctors attract over 20,000 new patients through their Upper Cervical Specific Marketing Programs.

Additionally, Dr. Davis is also actively involved as the Director of Public Relations for the National Upper Cervical Chiropractic Association (NUCCA) and the ICA's Council on Upper Cervical Care. Dr. Davis is also the host of the Upper Cervical Marketing Podcast. To learn more about Dr. Bill Davis and Upper Cervical Marketing go to www.uppercervicalmarketing.com.

CPSIA information can be obtained
at www.ICGtesting.com
Printed in the USA
BVHW090717011118
531456BV00002B/6/P

9 780692 154557